Cardiovascular Risk Factors in Pathology

Edited by Alaeddin Abukabda, Maria Suciu and Minodora Andor

Published in London, United Kingdom

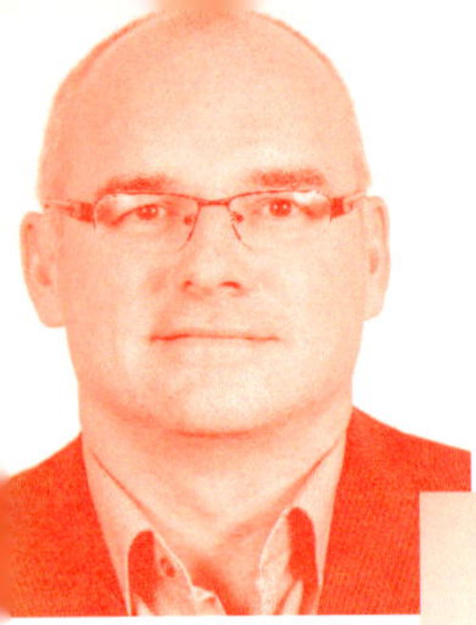
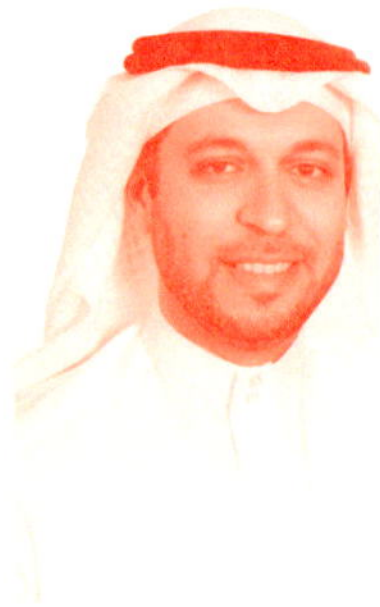
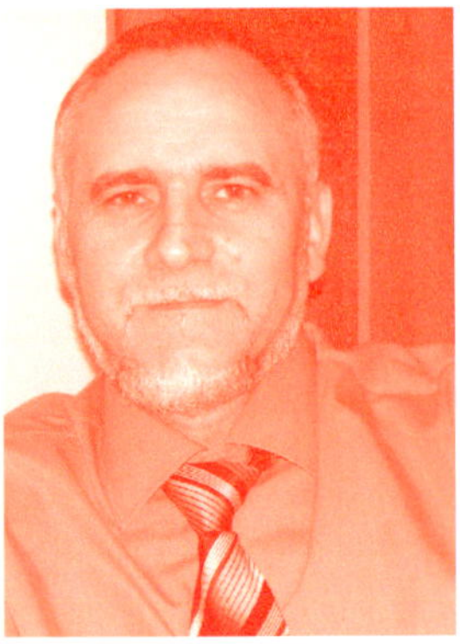
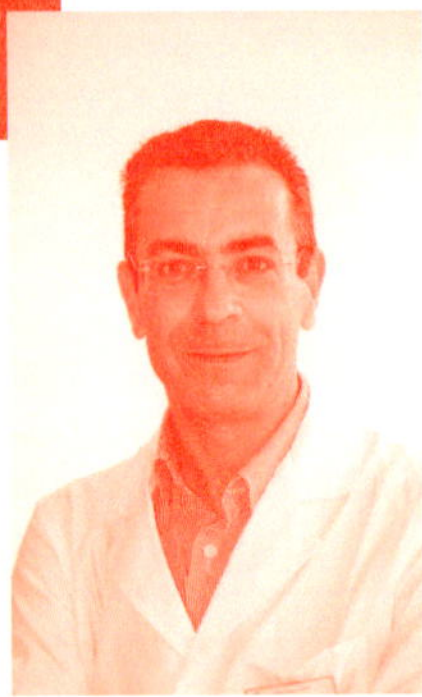
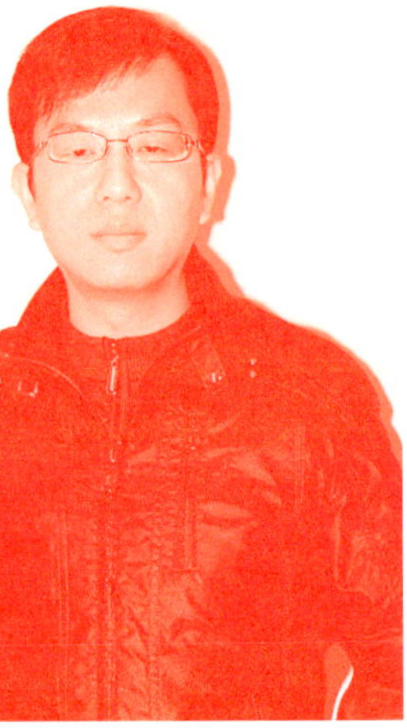
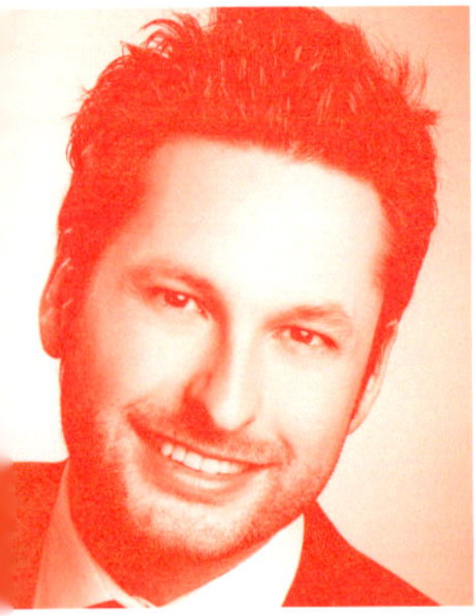
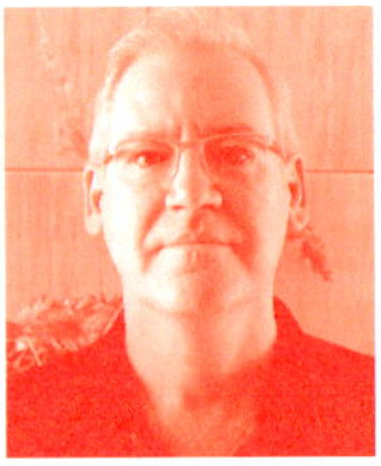

IntechOpen

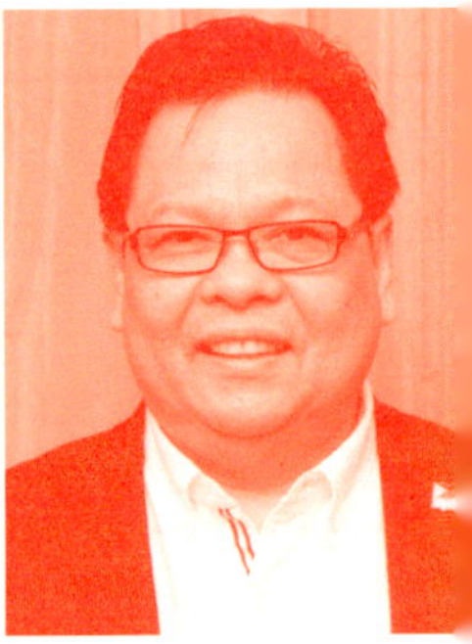
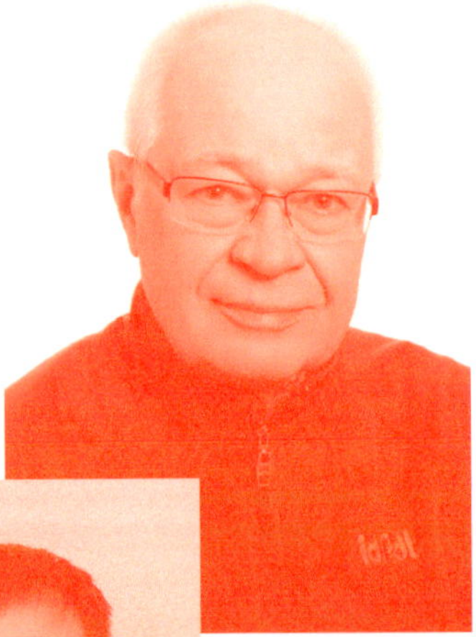
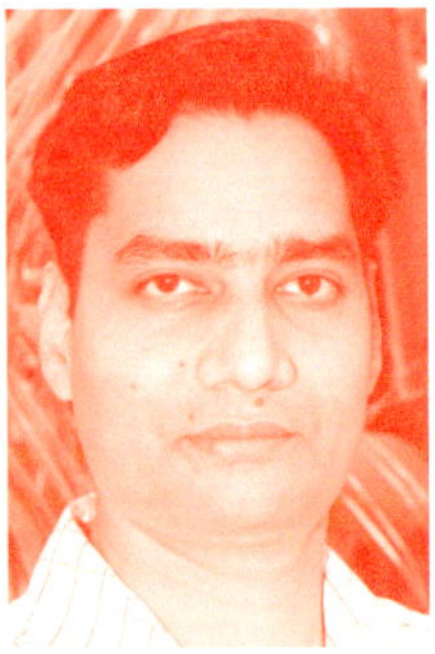
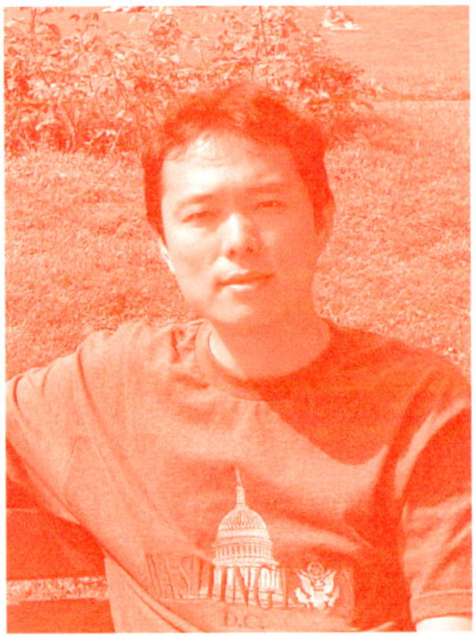
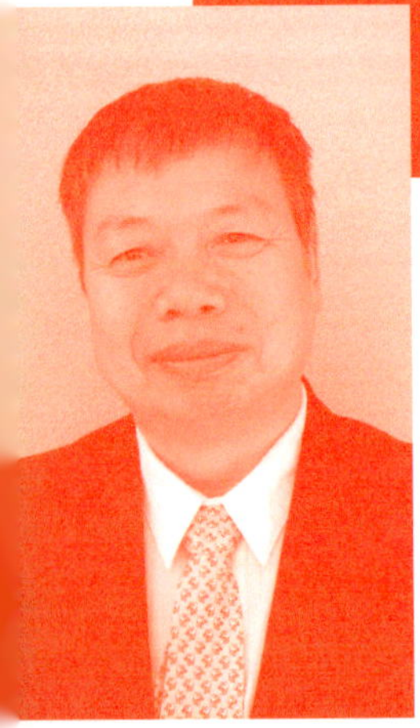
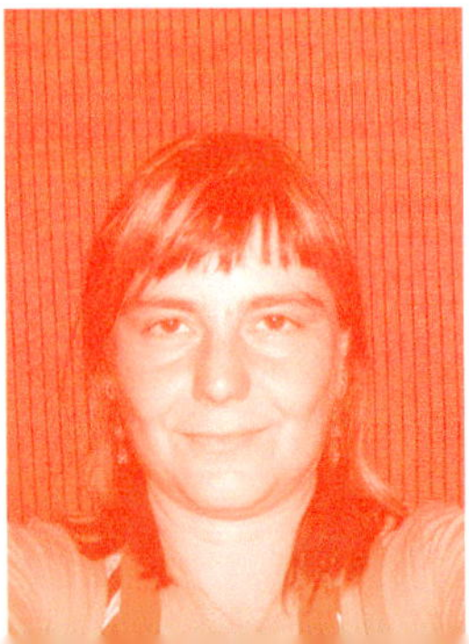

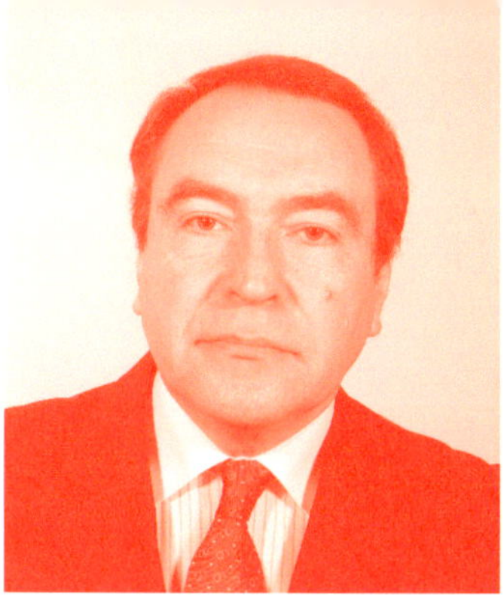
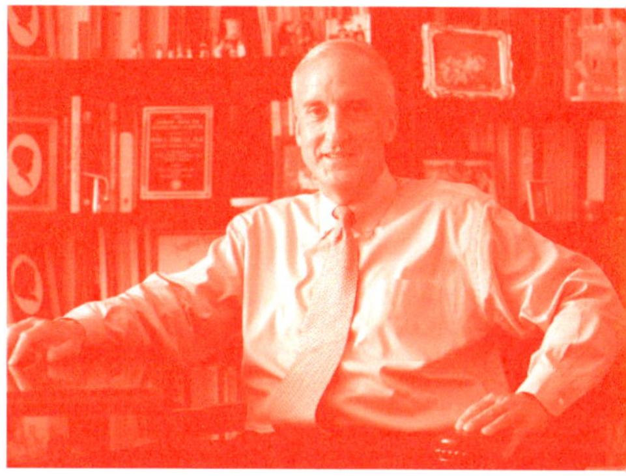
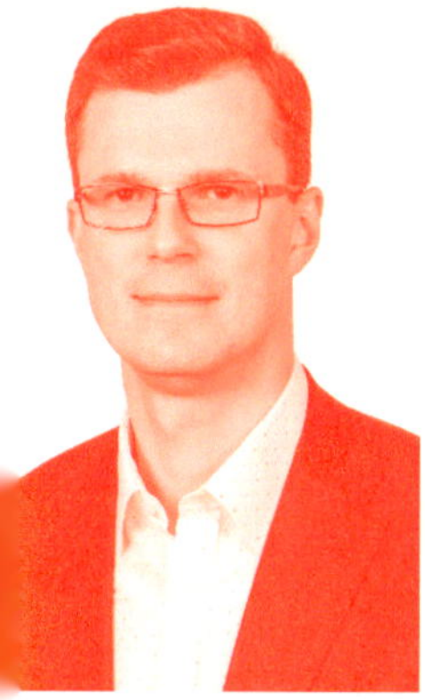
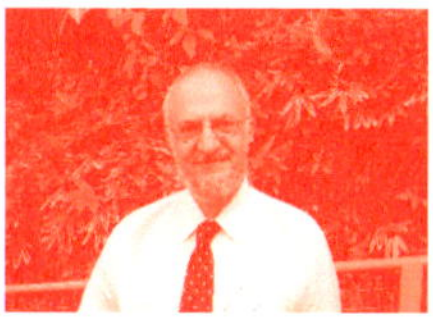
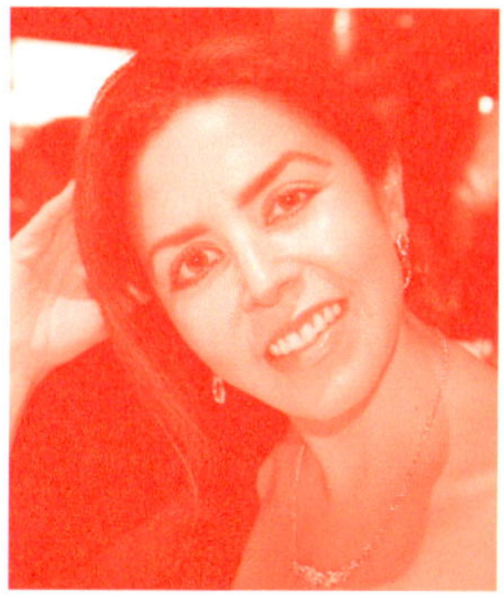

Supporting open minds since 2005

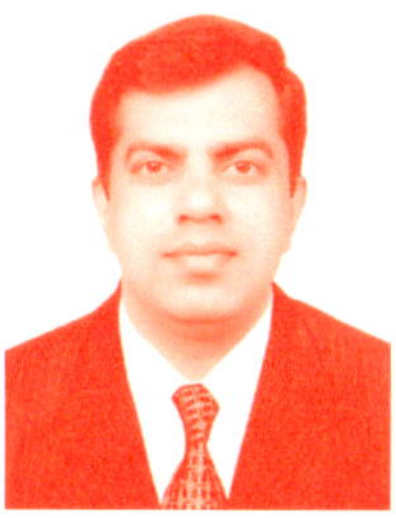
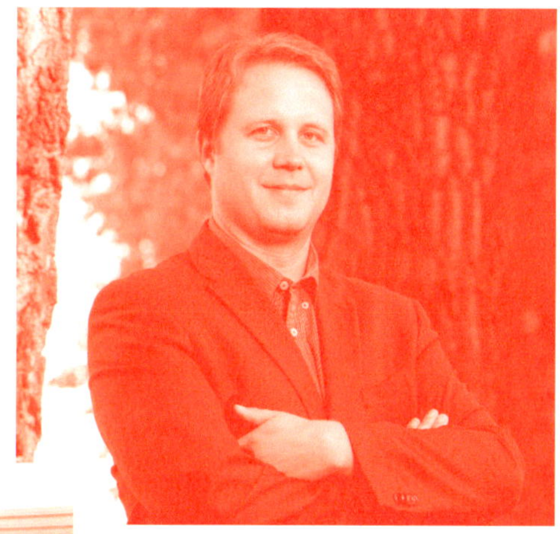
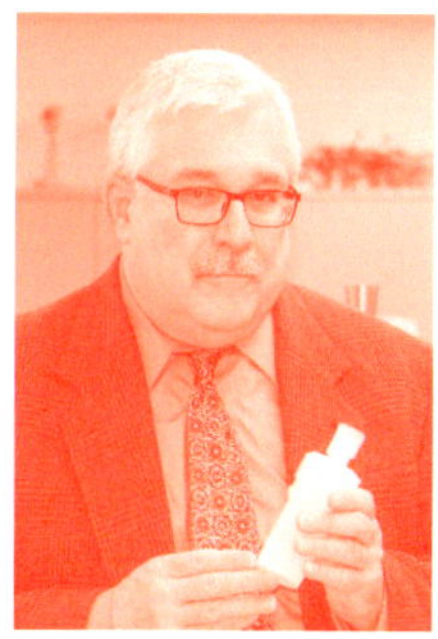
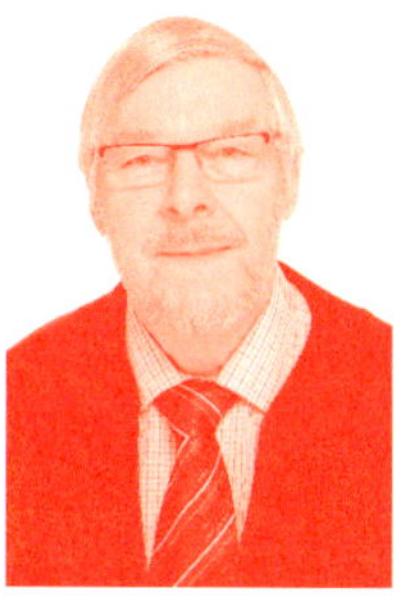
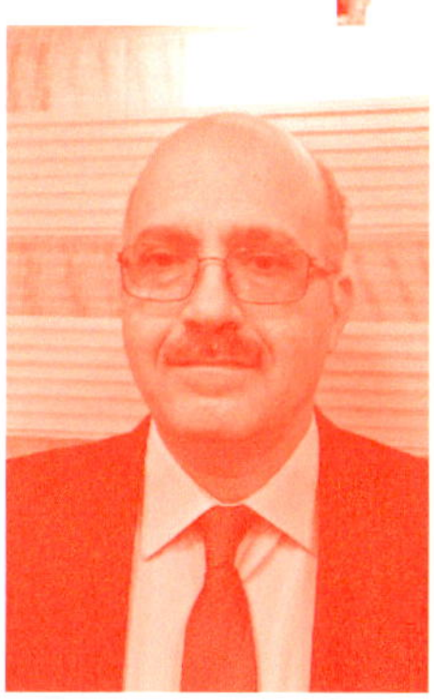
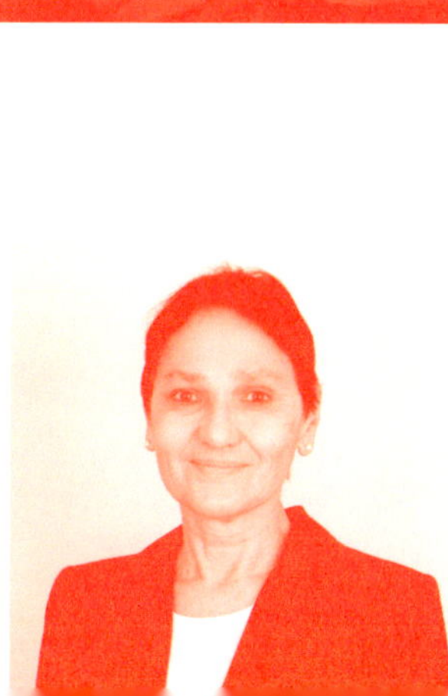
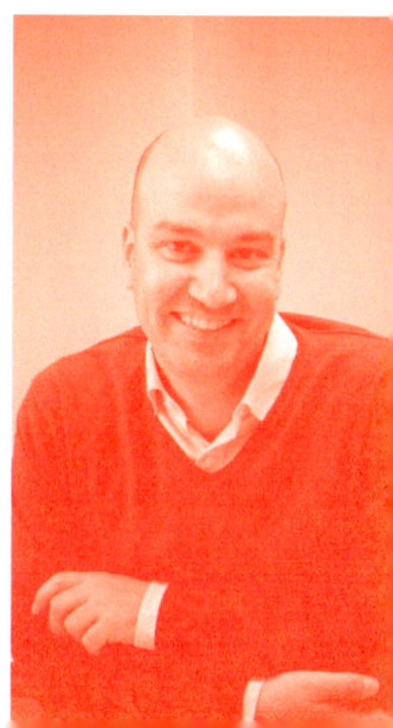

Cardiovascular Risk Factors in Pathology
http://dx.doi.org/10.5772/intechopen.73773
Edited by Alaeddin Abukabda, Maria Suciu and Minodora Andor

Contributors
Rajamma Mathew, Michael Patel, Robert Beasley, Daniel Braga, Andres Pirella, Brad Money, Brandon Olivieri, Adam Zybulewski, José López-Castro, Lucía Cid Conde, Ambika Pallikunnath Ashraf, Bhuvana Sunil, María Cristina Islas-Carbajal, Ana Rosa Rincon Sanchez, Cesar Arturo Nava Valdivia, Claudia Lisette Charles Niño, Vladimir O. Konstantinov

First published in London, United Kingdom, 2021 by IntechOpen
IntechOpen is the global imprint of INTECHOPEN LIMITED, registered in England and Wales, registration number: 11086078, 5 Princes Gate Court, London, SW7 2QJ, United Kingdom
Printed in Croatia

British Library Cataloguing-in-Publication Data
A catalogue record for this book is available from the British Library

Additional hard and PDF copies can be obtained from orders@intechopen.com

Cardiovascular Risk Factors in Pathology
Edited by Alaeddin Abukabda, Maria Suciu and Minodora Andor
p. cm.
Print ISBN 978-1-83881-949-1
Online ISBN 978-1-83881-950-7
eBook (PDF) ISBN 978-1-83881-951-4

For EU product safety concerns:
IN TECH d.o.o., Prolaz Marije Krucifikse Kozulić 3, 51000 Rijeka, Croatia, info@intechopen.com or visit our website at intechopen.com.

Meet the editors

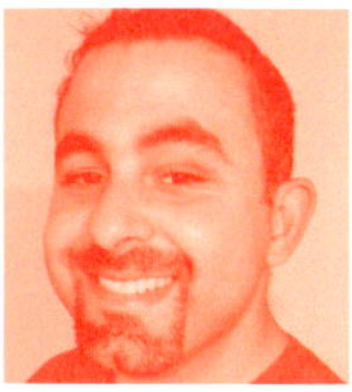

Dr. Abukabda graduated from Al Fateh Dental College, Libya, in 2007. He obtained a master`s degree in Molecular Biology from Clarion University, Pennsylvania, in 2011. He later obtained a Ph.D. in Cellular Physiology from West Virginia University in 2018 and a Certification in Biostatistics from the West Virginia University School of Public Health. In 2018, Dr. Abukabda worked as a postdoctoral research associate at the Vascular Medicine Institute at the University of Pittsburgh. He has been involved in the submission and writing of several National Institutes of Health (NIH) and National Science Foundation (NSF) grants and intramural seed grants. Dr. Abukabda has published and presented many papers in immunology, toxicology, and cardiovascular physiology. He has also served as a reviewer for many journals in his field of expertise.

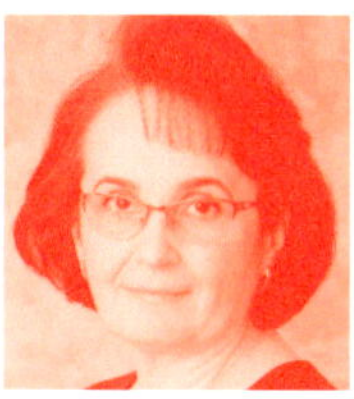

Dr. Maria Suciu is Assistant Professor of Pharmacology and Clinical Pharmacy in the Faculty of Pharmacy, "Victor Babes" University of Medicine and Pharmacy Timisoara, Romania. She received an MD in Family Medicine in 2003, an MPharm in 2011, and an MD in Cardiology in 2013, all from "Victor Babes" University of Medicine and Pharmacy Timisoara. Dr. Suciu has published one book chapter, eight scientific papers, and seventeen abstracts in international journals. She has also co-authored five books.

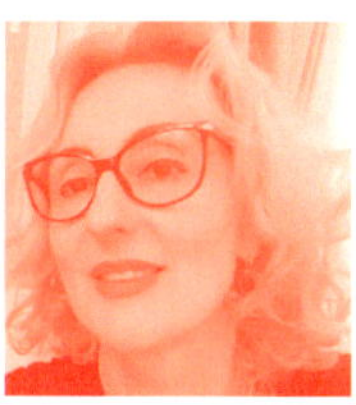

Assistant Professor Minodora Andor, Ph.D., graduated from the University of Medicine and Pharmacy "Victor Babes" Timisoara, Romania, in 1997. She completed her studies with a Ph.D. thesis addressing negative prognostic factors in the evolution of patients with acute myocardial infarction. Over the last twenty-three years, her personal research activity has focused on the study of cardiovascular pathology, particularly early diagnosis of atherosclerotic cardiovascular disease as well as the evolution of cardiac diseases in different pathological contexts. Her research interests include cardiovascular risk factors and endothelial dysfunction. Her professional work includes activities as a member of Timis College of Physicians and an expert with the European Commission for evaluating scientific projects within the Horizon 2020 frame.

Contents

Preface

The cardiovascular system is undoubtedly a key physiological regulator of the human body. Disruption of the delicate balance of its *milieu interieur* and dysfunction of its sophisticated functional cogs and wheels result in catastrophic events, which in most cases are irreversible. For these reasons, a deeper understanding of the pathophysiology of cardiovascular disease conditions is not only a must but is also a natural consequence of decades of evidence-based empirical scientific research.

The identification of microcirculation and more precisely of endothelial cells is a major milestone in cardiovascular physiology. Indeed, it is the editor's belief that all cardiovascular conditions can be traced back to some degree of microvascular endothelial dysfunction. However, notwithstanding the tremendous leaps and advancements undertaken by the scientific community, there is still a dire need for more effective therapeutic regimens. It is with this idea in mind that the current book has been shaped.

The scope of the current work is twofold. First, we provide a broad overview of the molecular mechanisms associated with relevant and significant cardiovascular conditions that continue to plague humanity. We discuss conditions such as pulmonary hypertension, familial hypercholesterolemia, aortic aneurysm, and dissection in depth. We also focus our attention on the pathogenesis of metabolic cardiomyopathy. While seemingly unrelated in etiology, these conditions have a recurring leitmotif: endothelial dysfunction. Second, we discuss potential and promising therapeutic avenues targeted at addressing these conditions. The overarching goal of this multifaceted and international work is to entice future and current members of the scientific community to direct their endeavors towards improving our current knowledge of cardiovascular disease conditions and curb their impact on our everyday lives.

Alaeddin Abukabda
Lake Erie College of Osteopathic Medicine,
Department of Physiology,
Erie, USA

Maria Suciu and Minodora Andor
Victor Babeș University of Medicine and Pharmacy,
Romania

Section 1

Mechanisms of Vascular Dysfunction

Chapter 1

Endothelial Dysfunction and Disruption in Pulmonary Hypertension

Rajamma Mathew

Abstract

A number of systemic diseases lead to pulmonary hypertension (PH), a serious disorder with a high morbidity and mortality rate. Irrespective of the underlying disease, endothelial dysfunction or disruption plays a key role in the initiation and progression of PH. Endothelial dysfunction and disruption result in impaired vascular relaxation response, activation of proliferative pathways leading to medial hypertrophy and PH. Endothelial cells (EC) play a crucial role in regulating vascular tone and maintaining homeostasis. Caveolin-1, a 21-22 kD membrane protein, interacts with a number of transducing factors and maintains them in a negative conformation. Disruption of EC results in endothelial caveolin-1 loss and reciprocal activation of proliferative pathways leading to PH, and the accompanying loss of PECAM1 and vascular endothelial cadherin results in barrier dysfunction. These changes lead to the irreversibility of PH. Hypoxia-induced PH is not accompanied by endothelial disruption or caveolin-1 loss but is associated with caveolin-1 dysfunction and the activation of proliferative pathways. Removal of hypoxic exposure results in the reversal of the disease. Thus, EC integrity is an important factor that determines irreversibility vs. reversibility of PH. This chapter will discuss normal EC function and the differences encountered in PH following EC disruption and EC dysfunction.

Keywords: caveolin-1, endothelial cells, membrane integrity, smooth muscle cells, pulmonary hypertension

1. Pulmonary hypertension

A number of systemic diseases such as cardiopulmonary, infectious, inflammatory and autoimmune diseases, hematological disorders, drug toxicity and several genetic mutations lead to pulmonary hypertension (PH), a devastating disease with a high morbidity and mortality rate. Based on clinical diagnosis, PH has been classified into five major groups that were updated in 2013 [1]. Group 1, labeled as pulmonary arterial hypertension (PAH), includes idiopathic and heritable PAH, PAH associated with congenital heart defect (CHD), connective tissue diseases, portal hypertension, HIV, schistosomiasis and drug-/toxin-induced PAH. In addition, mutation of several genes such as *BMPRII* (bone morphogenetic protein receptor type 2), *CAV1* (caveolin-1), *ENG* (endoglin), *SMAD9* (SMAD family member 9), *ACVRL1* (activin A receptor like type 1) and *KCNK3* (potassium two pore domain channel subfamily K member 3) are among the well-documented causes of PAH. Pulmonary veno-occlusive disease (PVOD)/pulmonary capillary hemangioma and persistent pulmonary hypertension of the newborn (PPHN) are included in Group 1 as subcategories 1′ and 1″, respectively. Recently, mutation of *EIF2AK4* (eukaryotic translation initiation factor 2a kinase 4) has been shown to be associated with PVOD and capillary hemangioma [2]. Included in Group 2 are PH associated with congenital and acquired left heart diseases; Group 3 comprises PH due to lung diseases and/or hypoxia. Group 4 includes chronic thromboembolic pulmonary hypertension (CTEPH). PH associated with hematological disorders, myeloproliferative diseases, splenectomy and a number of miscellaneous systemic and metabolic disorders is included in Group 5. Up until recently, the diagnosis of PAH was considered when the mean pulmonary artery pressure (PAP) of ≥25 mmHg, pulmonary capillary wedge pressure of ≤ 15 mmHg, and a pulmonary vascular resistance (PVR) of > 3 Wood units were observed at rest. During the 6th World Symposium on PH, the mean PAP of threshold was lowered to >20 mmHg and PVR was maintained as >3 Wood units [3]. These changes are based on the evaluation of 47 studies from 13 countries, which showed that independent of age the normal mean PAP rarely exceeded 20 mmHg [4]. The worldwide prevalence of PH is estimated to be 1%, increasing to 10% in patients older than 65 years of age. Globally, left heart diseases (Gr 2) and lung diseases (Gr 3) are considered the most common causes of PH. About 80% of patients are from developing countries; the common causes of PH in these patients are CHD, rheumatic heart disease and infection such as HIV and schistosomiasis. These patients tend to be younger than 65 years [5]. With modern therapy, the survival in patients with idiopathic and heritable PAH and PAH associated with anorexigen drugs has improved to 92%, 75% and 66% at 1, 3 and 5 years, respectively [6]. However, the underlying vascular changes remain progressive [7]. There is still a significant delay between the onset of symptoms and the final diagnosis. A recent retrospective study revealed a delay of 3.9 years between the onset of symptoms and the diagnosis of idiopathic PAH [8]. Thus, by the time the diagnosis is made, patients often have significant pulmonary vascular disease, which is a serious challenge to therapy. Interestingly, in an animal model of PH, significant disruption of endothelial cells and the activation of pro-proliferative pathways have been shown to occur before the onset of PH, indicating that the vascular pathology is already present by the time the symptoms appear [9].

The major causes of PH in children are CHD, PPHN, PH associated with disruption of normal pulmonary vascular and alveolar development in preterm infants, and congenital defects associated with hypoplasia of the lungs [10, 11]. A significant number of pediatric patients (>80%) have transient PH. These include resolution of PPHN and the majority of CHD cases that become free of PAH after the surgical correction of the defect [12]. However, preterm birth itself has an increased risk of developing PH even after adjusting for known factors such as heart and lung diseases, congenital diaphragmatic hernia and chromosomal abnormalities [13]. Furthermore, poor outcome has been reported in children with *BMPRII* mutation associated with idiopathic or heritable PAH [14]. Mutation of *TBX4* (T-box transcription factor 4 gene) is associated with skeletal, cardiac and neurologic defects. It also leads to a form of developmental lung disease that has been shown to be associated with severe PH during infancy and childhood [15]. It is worth noting that infants over the age of 2 years who had CHD exhibited increased pulmonary artery pressure and PVR even after surgical correction of the defect [16]. Pulmonary vascular lesions found in PAH associated with CHD are reported to be similar to what is found in idiopathic PAH [17]. However, the plexiform lesions in idiopathic PAH have monoclonal cell population, whereas Eisenmenger disease (PAH associated with CHD) displays polyclonal cells [18], indicating a distinct difference between two forms of PAH.

Endothelial cells (EC) play a key role in maintaining vascular homeostasis in response to various stimuli and regulate vascular tone, permeability, coagulation, inflammation through mediators such as nitric oxide (NO), endothelium-derived hyperpolarization factor (EDHF), endothelin-1 (ET1), cell adhesion molecules, cytokines and chemokines. Regardless of the underlying disease, endothelial dysfunction/disruption plays a key role in the pathogenesis of PH. The genetic and environmental factors act as an initial trigger leading to endothelial cell injury and impaired regeneration resulting in vascular remodeling and loss of small pulmonary arteries [19]. Endothelial dysfunction, impaired vascular dilatation, alterations in the expression of NO, ET1 and serotonin, increased expression of inflammatory cytokines and chemokines, loss of endothelial caveolin-1 and disordered proteolysis of extracellular matrix contribute to the pathogenesis of PAH [20, 21]. Increased expression of chemokines such as CX(3)C (fractalkine) and RANTES (CCL5) has been reported in PAH; importantly, both these chemokines are produced in EC [22, 23]. In sugen + hypoxia model (mice), the deletion of CCL5 resulted in reduction in PH via caveolin-1–dependent amplification of BMPR2 signaling. It stabilized surface caveolin-1, restored BMPR2 signaling and enhanced BMPR2 and caveolin-1 interaction [24]. This observation further supports the role for inflammation in PH. In addition, perivascular infiltration with inflammatory cells (T and B cells) is present in plexiform lesions [25, 26]. Increased expression of interleukin-1 (IL-1) and IL-6 occurs in human PAH and monocrotaline (MCT)-induced PH, and inhibition of IL-6 expression and bioactivity as a preventive measure results in the abrogation of MCT-induced PH [27, 28].

In addition to the imbalance of vasoactive mediators and vascular remodeling, abnormality in ion channels (Ca^{2+}, K^{+}) and growth factors such as VEGF, EGF, TGF beta, MMPs, BMPR2 and Notch1 has been implicated in pathophysiology of PAH, leading to vasoconstriction, abnormal remodeling and plexiform lesions [29]. Proliferative EC reveals increased expression of angiogenesis and survival-related molecules such as VEGF, VEGFR2, Hif-1 α, and 1β and reduced expression of p27/kip1. Signal transducer and activator of transcription (STAT3) is essential for cell proliferation and survival, and antiapoptotic function [30]. In the MCT model of PH, the loss of endothelial caveolin-1 was shown to be associated with reciprocal activation of STAT3 (PY-STAT3) and increased proliferating cell nuclear antigen (PCNA) [31]. Furthermore, EC in plexiform and concentric lesions exhibits increased expression of PY-STAT3 [32]. Importantly, the inhibition of STAT3 prevents neointima formation by inhibiting cell proliferation and promoting the apoptosis of neointimal SMC [33]. *BMPRII* mutations linked to PAH are associated with the activation of STAT3. Furthermore, BMPR2 deficiency promotes inflammatory response resulting in increased IL-6 levels and PY-STAT3 activation [34]. BMPR2, a cell surface receptor, is essential for differentiation and proliferation of EC and SMC. Without altering the *BMPRII* mRNA levels, miR-17/92 modulates BMPR2 protein levels. Importantly, IL-6 regulates the expression of miR-17/92 in human pulmonary arterial EC via STAT3 signaling. Persistent activation of STAT3 results in the upregulation of miR-20, which leads to the reduction in the expression of BMPR2 protein [35]. BMPR2 expression is decreased also in patients with heritable and idiopathic PAH, without associated mutation [36]. Importantly, levels of SMAD-specific E3 ubiquitin protein ligase 1 (Smurf1), a key negative regulator of BMPPR2, has been shown to be increased in hypoxia and MCT models of PH in rats [37]. Increased Smurf1 immunoreactivity has also been reported in EC and SMC in the explanted lungs from patients with PAH. Furthermore, Smurf1 deletion protects mice from sugen + hypoxia-induced PH [38]. Interestingly, elafin reverses obliterative changes in pulmonary arteries via elastase inhibition and caveolin-1–dependent amplification of BMPR2. In addition, elafin promotes angiogenesis via increasing interaction of BMPR2 and caveolin-1 via mediating stabilization of endothelial surface caveolin-1 [39].

Recent studies have shown the involvement of Notch1 signaling in PAH. Increased expression of Notch1 has been reported in the lungs of patients with IPAH and in rats with sugen + hypoxia-induced PH. Notch1 positively regulates EC proliferation by downregulating p21 and negatively regulating apoptosis via Bcl2 and survivin. *In-vitro* studies with human pulmonary arterial EC revealed increased expression of Notch1 during hypoxia exposure, and Notch1 downregulation decreased cell proliferation [40]. Furthermore, Notch1 under hypoxia contributes to increased proliferation, migration and survival in cancer cells [41]. Notch1 is essential for VEGF-induced proliferation, migration and survival of EC [42]. Thus, Notch1 plays a significant role in the pathogenesis of PH. However, Notch1 also plays a key role in vascular morphogenesis, EC quiescence, junction stability and vascular homeostasis. Reduction in Notch1 activity destabilizes cellular junction and triggers EC proliferation and results in the loss of arterial identity and incorporation of these cells into veins. Notch1 is sensitive to shear stress and it requires VEGFA and VEGFR2 for growth [43, 44]. Interestingly, Notch-mediated inhibition of proliferation requires phosphatase-tensin homolog (PTEN), a dual lipid/protein phosphatase. PTEN localization is cell cycle dependent, negatively regulates cell cycle progression and has a restrictive role on angiogenesis [45]. Recent studies have shown significant loss of PTEN concomitant with caveolin-1 dysfunction in hypoxia-induced PH [46]. Fibroblasts from idiopathic pulmonary fibrosis lungs exhibit low membrane PTEN associated with low membrane caveolin-1 levels, and overexpression of caveolin-1 restores membrane PTEN levels. PTEN contains a caveolin-1–binding motif and, in part, colocalizes in caveolae [47]. Thus, caveolin-1 expression determines the membrane PTEN levels through its binding sequence. Furthermore, PTEN has also been shown to negatively regulate STAT3 and its activation, and importantly, membrane localization of PTEN is considered responsible for the inactivation of STAT3 [48].

2. Endothelial cell function

EC forms a monolayer in contact with blood flow and mechanical forces and underlying SMC. It is a non-thrombogenic and a selective barrier to circulating macromolecules. Juxtaposition of EC and SMC facilitates cross talk, and EC maintains SMC in quiescent state. Myoendothelial gap junction plays an important role in Ca^{2+} exchange between EC and SMC. EC is crucial for delivery of O_2 and nutrients to underlying organs. EC maintains a balance between vasodilatation and vasoconstriction, apoptosis and cell proliferation, participate in immune and metabolic function, and maintain anticoagulant state [21, 49]. In addition, EC converts mechanical information into biological responses through mechanotransduction processes. EC adapts to mechanical inputs while maintaining crucial vascular barrier function. Failure of EC to adapt to changes has effects on vascular permeability, an important cause of vascular diseases [50].

2.1 Caveolae, caveolin-1 and cavin-1

Caveolae, a subset of specialized lipid rafts (50–100 nm), first described in 1950s by Palade [51] and Yamada [52], is found on plasma membranes of a variety of cell types including EC, SMC, fibroblasts and adipocytes. Caveolae are non-clathrin–coated plasma membrane vesicles (50–100 nm) enriched in glycosphingolipids, cholesterol, sphingomyelin and lipid-anchored membrane proteins. They form an important signaling platform that compartmentalizes and integrates a number of signaling molecules and allows cross talk between different signaling pathways, and mediates and integrates signaling events at the cell surface. EC contains 5000–10,000 caveolae per cell [53]. In addition, caveolae act as plasma membrane sensors and respond to stress. Caveolae flatten in response to membrane stretch. The flattening is a protective mechanism; it buffers the membrane and prevents its rupture [54, 55]. Caveolin-1 is a major protein (21–22 kDa) constituent of caveolae that maintains the shape of caveolae; EC has the highest levels of caveolin-1 [56]. Caveolin-1 is involved in multiple cellular processes such as molecular transport, cell proliferation, adhesion, migration and signal transduction. Caveolin-1 has an integral role in endocytosis. However, overexpression of caveolin-1 inhibits endocytosis [57, 58]. Caveolin-1 is synthesized in endoplasmic reticulum and then transported to Golgi complex. During its biosynthesis, it is associated with lipid rafts and become detergent resistant. From a structural standpoint, caveolin-1 contains a hairpin loop structure and three palmitoylation sites and a scaffolding domain that facilitates interaction with the plasma membrane [59, 60]. Caveolin-1 functions through protein-protein interaction and regulates and stabilizes several proteins including Src family of kinases, G proteins (α-subunits), G protein-coupled receptors, H-Ras, PKC, endothelial NO synthase (eNOS), integrins, and growth factor receptors such as VEGFR2, EGFR and PDGFR in an inhibitory conformation. Importantly, a 20-amino acid membrane proximal region of the cytosolic amino-terminal domain, termed caveolin-scaffolding domain (residue 82–101), is sufficient to mediate these interactions [61, 62]. Caveolin-1 also functions as a suppressor of cytokine signaling (SOCS), the family of proteins that are upregulated by cytokines and that in turn inhibit cytokine signaling via modulating JAK-STAT pathway [63]. Caveolin-2 is present associated with caveolin-1 in all cell types. It requires caveolin-1 for its transport from Golgi body to the plasma membrane. Caveolin-2 is not necessary for caveolae formation or caveolar localization of caveolin-1, but the coexpression results in a more efficient formation of caveolae [64]. In the absence of caveolin-1, caveolin-2 is degraded, and the decreased expression of caveolin-2 promotes increased cell proliferation [65, 66]. Furthermore, caveolin-2 knockout mice display increased proliferation of endothelial cells, hyper-cellular lung parenchyma and cell cycle progression [67].

In addition to caveolin-1, caveolae require polymerase 1 and transcript release factor (PTRF) also known as cavin-1. It is an essential component of caveolae; it regulates membrane curvature by stabilizing caveolin-1 in caveolae. The loss of cavin-1 results in the loss of caveolae and the release of caveolin-1 into the plasma membrane. Importantly, caveolin-1 is required for cavin-1 recruitment to plasma membrane [68, 69]. Loss of caveolin-1 is accompanied by a marked loss of caveolin-2 and partial reduction in cavin-1 expression in the lungs. The re-expression of caveolin-1 rescues both caveolin-2 and cavin-1 [70]. In a carotid artery-injury model, the local loss of cavin-1 is reported to promote neointima formation. Furthermore, in cultured vascular SMC, the overexpression of cavin-1 suppresses SMC proliferation and migration, whereas its inhibition promotes cell proliferation and migration [71]. Cavin-1 knockout mice display lung pathological changes such as remodeled pulmonary vessels, PH and right ventricular hypertrophy. In addition, these mice have altered metabolic phenotype with insulin resistance [72, 73].

Recent studies have shown other accessory proteins required in caveolae biogenesis. The accessory protein pacsin2 also known as syndapin2 contains F-BAR domain associated with generation and maintenance of caveolae. It partially colocalizes with caveolin-1 at plasma membrane level. Loss of pacsin2 function results in the loss of caveolae and accumulation of caveolin-1 within the plasma membrane. Interestingly, overexpression of F-BAR domain can cause loss of caveolae. Another protein EH 15 homology domain 2 (EHD2) is present in caveolae, and it binds to pacsin2 that partially colocalizes with caveolin-1. It is a dynamin-related ATPase that confines caveolae to cell surface. Furthermore, regulation of EHD2 oligomerization in a membrane-bound state is crucial in order to restrict caveolar dynamics in cells [74, 75]. Importantly, caveolar coat controls a large number of signaling circuits; a defect in any of these pathways can lead to several systemic diseases such as vascular dysfunction, cardiomyopathy, cancer, muscular dystrophy and lipodystrophy [76].

The role of caveolin-1 is well established in the pathogenesis of PH. Caveolin-1 knockout mice are viable but have dysregulated NO synthesis, impaired NO and Ca^{2+} signaling, cell proliferation, increased vascular permeability accompanied by cardiomyopathy and PH. Reconstituting endothelial caveolin-1 has been shown to recover dysregulated NO synthesis, cardiomyopathy and PH [77, 78]. In addition, caveolin-1 knockout mice exhibit low-grade systemic pro-inflammatory status and moderately increased IL-6 and TNFα levels [79]. EC-specific *CAV1* knockout mice and LPS-treated wild-type mice exhibit reduced BMPR2 expression and eNOS uncoupling, accompanied by increased TGF-β–promoted TGFβRI-dependent SMAD-2/3 phosphorylation. In addition, human lung sections from patients with ARDS reveal reduced endothelial caveolin-1 expression, increased TGF-β levels and severe pulmonary vascular remodeling. These results further support the view that the loss of endothelial caveolin-1 promotes pulmonary vascular remodeling in inflamed lungs via oxidative stress-mediated reduction in BMPR2 expression [80]. Furthermore, endothelial dysfunction during inflammation leads to endothelium-mesenchymal transition (End MT). These cells lose endothelial characteristics and acquire mesenchymal phenotypes and express mesenchymal specific markers such as smooth muscle α-actin, fibroblast-specific protein 1 and Notch1 [81]. In addition, caveolin-1 is a determinant of oxidative stress and is a regulator of metabolic switch and autophagy [82].

2.2 Vascular relaxation

NO, EDHF and prostacyclin (PGI2) induce endothelium-dependent vascular relaxation. NO is produced by eNOS via its action on L-arginine and oxygen. NO activates guanylate cyclase, which catalyzes the conversion of guanosine triphosphate to cyclic guanylate monophosphate. eNOS expressed in endothelial cells and cardiac myocytes is targeted to caveolae. It directly binds to caveolin-1 scaffolding domain and is held in an inhibitory state. This interaction prevents eNOS activation leading to inappropriate NO production under basal conditions. The eNOS/caveolin-1 regulatory cycle is a reversible protein-protein interaction controlled by Ca^{2+}/calmodulin and by enzyme palmitoylation. Increase in intracellular Ca^{2+} with calmodulin disrupts the caveolin-1/eNOS complex resulting in eNOS activation and NO production leading to vascular relaxation. Calmodulin is a direct allosteric competitor promoting the caveolin-1 and eNOS dissociation. Heat shock protein (HSP) 90 binds to eNOS in Ca^{2+}/calmodulin-dependent manner and it reduces the inhibitory effects of caveolin scaffolding domain on eNOS, thus promoting eNOS activation [83–85]. Furthermore, increase in vascular flow and pressure rapidly activates caveolar eNOS with its dissociation from caveolin-1 and association with calmodulin [86]. Thus, caveolin-1 and eNOS have a dynamic relationship. Importantly, caveolin-1 contained within non-caveolar lipid rafts fails to exert its inhibitory effect on eNOS [87]. The loss of endothelial caveolin-1 leads to eNOS uncoupling, oxidative stress and endothelial injury [88]. Interestingly, under conditions of stress, caveolin-1 increases eNOS trafficking in plasma membrane and primes eNOS for flow-mediated activation. Caveolin-1 plays a positive role in shear-induced eNOS activation by targeting eNOS to plasma membrane. Importantly, the coupling of flow stimulus to activate eNOS is lost in the absence of caveolin-1 and caveolae. Thus, caveolin-1 exerts dual role of post-translational regulation of eNOS activity [89]. In addition, caveolin-1 plays a critical role in VEGFR2 stimulation and downstream mediators of angiogenesis, but higher levels of caveolin-1 repress this function [90]. Interestingly, EC migration, tube formation and angiogenesis are impaired both in caveolin-1 and eNOS knockout mice but are fully restored by double knockout [91].

The transient receptor potential (TRP) channels are the link between caveolae and EDHF. TRP channels facilitating the capacitive Ca^{2+} entry directly interact with caveolin-1 in EC. Ca^{2+}-activated K^+ channels play a key role in endothelium-dependent hyperpolarization and vascular tone regulation. Absence of caveolin-1 impairs Ca^{2+} homeostasis in EC and decreases the activity of TPRV4 cation channels that participate in NO and EDHF activation. Caveolin-1 is required for EDHF-related relaxation, modulating TRPV4 and connexins. Caveolin-1 knockout arteries exhibit fewer gap junctions and altered myoendothelial communication. Furthermore, caveolin-1 deficiency is associated with impaired EDHF-mediated vascular relaxation in response to shear stress and acetylcholine [92–94]. Colocalization of PGI2 synthase and caveolin-1 regulates angiogenesis [95]. Thus, caveolin-1 interacts with relaxing factors to maintain homeostasis.

2.3 Barrier function

Endothelial barrier controls the passage of fluids, nutrients and cells through vascular wall. Glycocalyx coats the luminal surface of EC and forms an important barrier. It modulates permeability, prevents leukocyte and platelet adhesion to EC, serves as an anti-inflammatory, anti-adhesive and anti-coagulant barrier, and allows selective permeability. In addition, it mediates mechanotransduction of shear stress. Under normal conditions, the apoptosis rate in EC is very low, but the activated EC exhibits a reduction in the EC surface layer, the glycocalyx, and an increased rate of apoptosis [96, 97]. Disturbed flow has been shown to inhibit glycocalyx expression as well as to reduce caveolin-1 expression in systemic arterial EC [98]. Inflammatory mediators lead to the disruption of glycocalyx resulting in the weakening of vascular protection. Integrity of vascular glycocalyx is inversely related to the degree of inflammation. Inflammatory mediators lead to the loss of glycocalyx resulting in the weakening of vascular protection. Furthermore, destruction of glycocalyx has been reported in the MCT model of PH [99].

Ca^{2+}-dependent vascular endothelial cadherin (VE-Cad) and its associated catenins control cell-cell adhesion and paracellular barrier function and are important for the tight junction complexes. VE-Cad is tissue specific for EC and is expressed at the intercellular clefts and mediates cell-cell adhesion, maintains barrier function, and contributes to the inhibition of cell growth. Association of caveolin-1 and VE-Cad catenin complex is essential for barrier function [100–102]. Depletion of caveolin-1 reduces VE-Cad levels and facilitates endothelial cell permeability [103]. Furthermore, VE-Cad interacts with various growth receptors, regulates endothelial proliferative signaling and mediates contact inhibition of cell growth [104, 105]. In adult EC, VE-Cad and VEGFR2 are physically linked. This maintains VEGFR2 stable and prevents its endocytosis. VEGF-induced permeability is facilitated by decoupling of VE-Cad and VEGFR2 [106]. Loss of VE-Cad and PECAM1 has been shown to occur in the MCT-induced PH [31, 107]. PECAM-1 supports EC integrity and maintains barrier function [108]. Importantly, BMPR2 also plays a role in maintaining vascular integrity by dampening inflammatory signals in pulmonary vasculature [109].

3. Endothelial disruption/dysfunction

Vascular injury from different conditions such as inflammation, hypoxia, increased flow and pressure, and shear stress leads to endothelial dysfunction. Injury can lead to disruption of EC and endothelial caveolin-1 loss or endothelial dysfunction without EC disruption. Both lead to the activation of proliferative pathways, vascular remodeling and PH [96, 110]. Recent studies have shown the loss of myocyte enhancer factor 2 (MEF2) in dysfunctional EC from PAH patients. MEF2 regulates a number of transcription factors involved in pulmonary vascular homeostasis [111]. Furthermore, these dysfunctional ECs exhibit increased production of leptin, and SMCs overexpress leptin receptor contributing to SMC proliferation [112]. In addition, pulmonary arterial ECs from PAH patients have been shown to produce increased FGF2 leading to increased proliferation and survival response by constitutive activation of ERK1/2 and decreased apoptosis associated with the activation of Bcl2 and Bcl-xL. It is thought that FGF2 in PAH may contribute to abnormal EC phenotype [113]. Furthermore, there is evidence that pro-inflammatory cytokine macrophage migration inhibitory factor and its receptor CD74 are markedly increased in idiopathic PAH, which may contribute to pro-inflammatory phenotype of EC [114].

3.1 EC disruption and pulmonary hypertension

Endothelial disruption accompanied by the loss of endothelial caveolin-1 has been reported in several forms of experimental models of PH such as MCT, myocardial infarction and sugen + hypoxia [31, 115, 116]. In the MCT model, progressive loss of endothelial caveolin-1 and reciprocal activation of proliferative and anti-apoptotic pathways such as PY-STAT3 and Bcl-xL occur before the onset of PH. Loss of other membrane proteins such as PECAM-1, Tie2 and soluble guanylate cyclase (α and β) occurs in tandem with caveolin-1 loss indicating extensive disruption of endothelial cell membrane. At 2 weeks, a further loss of endothelial caveolin-1 is accompanied by the loss of cytosolic proteins such as HSP90 and IκB-α and increased pulmonary artery pressure. However, at this stage, eNOS expression is relatively well preserved. In the presence of significant loss of endothelial caveolin-1 and HSP90, eNOS gets uncoupled resulting in an increased production of reactive oxygen species (ROS). By 3 and 4 weeks, there is a significant reduction in eNOS levels, leading to normalization of ROS levels [9, 31, 117]. At 4 weeks post-MCT, extensive endothelial caveolin-1 loss is accompanied by the loss of von Willebrand factor (vWF) in 29% of the arteries; and 23% of arteries exhibit enhanced expression of caveolin-1 in SMC. Enhanced expression of caveolin-1 in SMC occurs only in the arteries with extensive endothelial caveolin-1 and vWF loss. At this stage, the expression of total caveolin-1 in the lungs remains low. In addition, there is a progressive increase in MMP2 expression and activation [117]. The rescue of endothelial caveolin-1 as a preventive measure abrogates MCT-induced PH, but once the PH is established, the treatment does not alter the progression of the disease [118–120]. Exposing MCT-treated rats to hypoxia accelerates the disease process, and by 4 weeks, extensive endothelial disruption and endothelial caveolin-1 loss are accompanied by enhanced expression of caveolin-1 in SMC in 61% of the arteries, near normalization of lung caveolin-1 expression, and neointima formation. Importantly, neointimal cells exhibit low to no caveolin-1 expression [121, 122]. Extensive loss of endothelial caveolin-1, enhanced expression of caveolin-1 in SMC and neointima formation are also observed in idiopathic and hereditary PAH, PAH associated with CHD and drug toxicity [122–125]. In *in-vitro* studies, pulmonary arterial SMCs from idiopathic PAH exhibit increased caveolin-1 expression accompanied by increased capacitive Ca^{2+} entry and DNA synthesis, which could be abrogated by silencing caveolin-1 [125]. Loss of EC exposes SMC to direct pressure and shear stress, which is likely to result in flattening of caveolae leading to displacement of caveolin-1 to non-caveolar site on the plasma membrane. Recently, it has been shown that in the MCT + hypoxia model, at 4 weeks, the extensive loss of endothelial caveolin-1 as well as VE-Cad loss and enhanced expression of caveolin-1 in SMC are accompanied by cavin-1 loss, tyrosine phosphorylation of caveolin-1 and neointima formation. Loss of VE-Cad is indicative of loss of EC attachment to the junction [126]. Interestingly, p-caveolin-1 in cancer has been shown to make cells pro-migratory [127, 128]. As PH progresses, SMC phenotype changes from contractile to synthetic, facilitating cell migration, and neointima formation resulting in arterial occlusion. Neointima formation leads to the irreversibility of the disease [129]. In addition, increasing pulmonary blood flow either by pneumonectomy or by a shunt procedure (left subclavian and pulmonary artery) in rats treated with MCT leads to the development of neointimal lesions. Pneumonectomy or shunt alone does not lead to neointima formation [130, 131]. Furthermore, in children with significant left to right cardiac shunt, reversal of pulmonary vascular changes were seen after they underwent pulmonary artery banding to restrict the pulmonary flow. Medial hypertrophy and early intimal changes seem reversible, but not during the later stages [132, 133]. These studies demonstrate that EC injury and disruption associated with increased flow or pressure play an important role in determining the pattern of pulmonary vascular remodeling.

Apoptosis of EC in PAH is followed by proliferation of antiapoptotic EC. This concept has been confirmed in *in-vitro* studies. Sugen (VEGFR antagonist) causes initial apoptosis, and the surviving cells become hyperproliferative [134]. Importantly, increased levels of circulating EC (CEC) have been reported in PAH, and 50% of these cells expressed CD36, a marker of microvascular origin, and 25% exhibited E selectin, a marker of EC activation [135]. In children with CHD and PAH, the increased levels of CEC are reported to be associated with worse prognosis. Pulmonary ECs exhibited high expression of antiapoptotic protein Bcl-2 in cases of irreversible PAH but not in cases of reversible PAH, or in controls. Interestingly, intimal proliferation was observed only in irreversible PAH cases, but not in the reversible PAH [136, 137]. In addition, increased vWF levels in patients with PAH were reported to be associated with worse survival [138]. Interestingly, increased CEC levels were observed in PAH, but not in CTEPH [139]. These studies strongly support the view that the disruption and loss of EC are associated with severe PAH and poor prognosis.

Endothelial mesenchymal transition (EndMT) is a process by which ECs exhibit phenotype alteration. These cells lose endothelial characteristics and acquire the properties of myofibroblasts or mesenchymal cells. They exhibit loss of PECAM-1 and VE-Cad, in addition to caveolin-1, and express smooth muscle α-actin, fibroblast-specific protein 1 and Notch1. PECAM-1 and VE-Cad support EC integrity and junctional stability and maintain barrier function. Thus, their loss leads to the loss of barrier function and junction stability. These transformed ECs also acquire pro-inflammatory phenotype and are primed for proliferation, migration and tissue generation [81, 140]. Neointimal cells exhibit low levels of caveolin-1, but normal eNOS expression in the experimental model of PH and also in human PAH [96, 122], and sustained NO production has been shown to degrade caveolin-1 [141]. Importantly, caveolin-1 deficiency has been shown to induce spontaneous EndMT in pulmonary EC [142]. EndMT plays an important role in vascular remodeling, and it is also linked to the loss of BMPR2 in PH [143–145]. Furthermore, TGFβ1 plays a significant role in EndMT [146]. In addition, endothelial caveolin-1 depletion leads to eNOS uncoupling and oxidative stress that switches from BMPR2 signaling to TGFβR1 and thus may promote EndMT [80]. Plexogenic lesions contain increased VEGFA and VEGFR expression indicating misguided angiogenesis involving cells of EC origin. EC dysfunction in PAH model is shown to act through DNA methylation, histone protein modification and non-coding RNA [19]. Thus, the initial apoptosis followed by the proliferation of dysfunctional and antiapoptotic EC leads to deregulation of a number of pathways resulting in neointima and plexiform lesion formation and irreversible PAH.

3.2 EC dysfunction without EC disruption and pulmonary hypertension

Exposure to acute hypoxia results in pulmonary arterial contraction and elevated pulmonary artery pressure, while sustained hypoxia leads to pulmonary vascular remodeling [147]. Hypoxia impairs endothelium-dependent relaxation response [148, 149]. In the MCT model of PH, the progressive loss of endothelial caveolin-1 is accompanied by a significant reduction in the expression of HSP90 (2 weeks post-MCT) and eNOS (3 weeks post-MCT) [9]. However, hypoxia does not alter the protein expression of caveolin-1, eNOS or HSP90 in the lungs. During hypoxia, caveolin-1 and eNOS have been shown to form a tight complex *in vivo* and *in vitro*, resulting in their dysfunction [110, 150]. Normally, in response to Ca^{2+} agonists, eNOS dissociates from caveolin-1 and binds to HSP90. Ca^{2+} activated calmodulin further aids in recruitment of HSP90, thus facilitating the release of eNOS from caveolin-1 [151]. However, hypoxia disrupts eNOS/HSP90 binding [152]. Furthermore, normally functioning caveolin-1 is required for the plasma membrane localization of TRPC4 and endothelial Ca^{2+} entry [153], and introduction of caveolin-1 scaffolding domain restores Ca^{2+} entry during chronic hypoxia [154]. Thus, the hypoxia-induced caveolin-1 and eNOS complex formation may in part be responsible for the deregulation of Ca^{2+} entry and disruption of HSP90/eNOS binding leading to impaired vascular relaxation. Statins have been shown to disrupt hypoxia-induced abnormal coupling of eNOS and caveolin-1, thus restoring eNOS function and attenuating hypoxia-induced PH [155]. Recent studies of hypoxia-induced PH in rats and cows showed no disruption of EC or any alterations in the expression of caveolin-1, VE-Cad or vWF [46, 126]. Not surprisingly, there was no enhanced expression of caveolin-1 in SMC as seen in the MCT model. However, there was evidence of caveolin-1 dysfunction, such as the activation of proliferative pathways such as PY-STAT3, β-catenin and pERK1/2, and a loss of PTEN. PTEN contains a Cav-1–binding motif and, in part, colocalizes in caveolae. Caveolin-1 determines the membrane PTEN levels through its binding sequence. The loss of PTEN during hypoxia further confirms caveolin-1 dysfunction [46].

People living at high altitude develop PH and right ventricular hypertrophy as an adaptive mechanism. Upon return to sea level, PH reverts to normal slowly [156]. These observations suggest that the absence of physical disruption of EC observed in the hypoxia model may be the reason why hypoxia-induced PH is reversible. Although hypoxia plays a role, inflammation and endothelial dysfunction are important factors that determine the development of PH in chronic obstructive pulmonary disease (COPD). The outflow obstruction in COPD results from inflammatory processes affecting airways, lung parenchyma and pulmonary vasculature. PH in COPD can develop independently of underlying parenchymal destruction and loss of lung vessels [157, 158]. Endothelial dysfunction has been observed in mild cases of COPD, and the loss of endothelium-dependent relaxation in the pulmonary vasculature correlates with the severity of the disease [159]. Importantly, the loss of endothelial caveolin-1 accompanied by enhanced expression of caveolin-1 in SMC is reported in COPD associated with PH. COPD without PH had preserved endothelial caveolin-1 [160]. In addition, severe pulmonary arterial lesions such as plexiform and angiomatoid lesions have been documented in explanted lungs after transplantation in COPD associated with severe PH. These lesions were similar to what are seen in IPAH [161]. In infants with respiratory distress syndrome, despite significantly elevated pulmonary artery pressure and significant medial thickening, pulmonary arteries exhibit well-preserved endothelial caveolin-1, without any evidence of EC disruption or enhanced expression of Cav-1 in SMC. In contrast, loss of endothelial Cav-1 and disruption/loss of EC coupled with enhanced expression of Cav-1 in SMC were observed in infants with bronchopulmonary dysplasia and associated inflammation [123]. These results indicate that irrespective of the underlying disease, EC disruption leads to the loss of endothelial caveolin-1 and subsequent enhanced expression of Cav-1 in SMC, followed by neointima formation and irreversible PH. Thus, the EC disruption puts the patients at a higher risk of developing irreversible PH.

4. Conclusions

Under normal conditions, ECs play a key role in maintaining SMCs in quiescent state and vascular homeostasis. Caveolin-1, a major protein constituent of caveolae on the cell membrane, regulates multiple cellular processes including inflammation, molecular transport, cell proliferation, adhesion, migration and signal transduction. Caveolin-1 interacts with protein molecules that are in or are recruited to caveolae and maintains them in inhibitory confirmation. Endothelial caveolin-1 loss and caveolin-1 dysfunction lead to PH.

4.1 EC disruption and caveolin-1 loss

Injury such as inflammation, increased pulmonary blood flow associated with increased pressure, drugs and toxins can cause endothelial disruption, which is usually progressive. Endothelial disruption leads to the progressive loss of endothelial membrane proteins including caveolin-1, PECAM-1 and VE-Cad. These alterations lead to deregulation of multiple pathways. As depicted in **Figure 1**, (a) the loss of caveolin-1 is accompanied by reciprocal activation of proliferative and antiapoptotic pathways leading to SMC hypertrophy and proliferation. (b) Further loss of EC exposes SMCs to direct pressure resulting in enhanced expression of caveolin-1 in SMCs. Tyrosine phosphorylated caveolin-1 could alter the phenotype and facilitate cell migration leading to neointima formation. (c) Loss of PECAM-1 and VE-Cad results in the loss of barrier function and junction stability. These alterations lead to EndMT. These cells lose endothelial properties and acquire pro-inflammatory phenotype and are primed for proliferation, migration and tissue generation and participate in neointima formation, thus leading to irreversible PH.

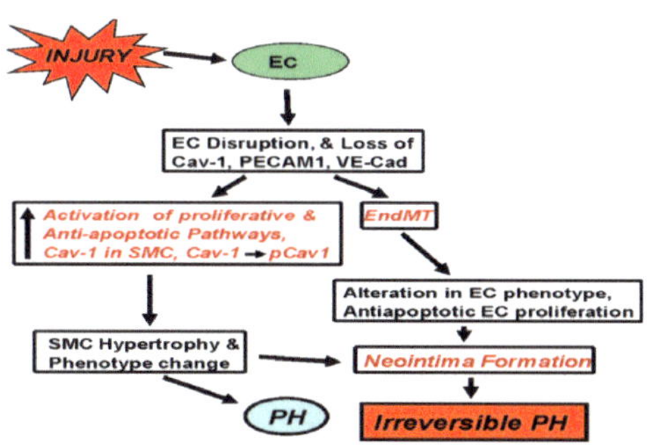

Figure 1.
This figure depicts the pathway leading from endothelial cell disruption to irreversible PH. Cav-1 = caveolin-1, EC = endothelial cells, EndMT = endothelial mesenchymal transformation, PECAM-1 = platelet endothelial cell adhesion molecule 1, pCav-1 = tyrosine phosphorylated caveolin-1, PH = pulmonary hypertension, SMC = smooth muscle cells.

4.2 EC and caveolin-1 dysfunction

Hypoxia exposure to EC leads to a tight complex formation between caveolin-1 and eNOS, resulting in the dysfunction of both factors (**Figure 2**). Importantly, there is no EC disruption or the loss of caveolin-1 or any other membrane proteins. Since there is no loss of EC, medial layer is not exposed to shear stress and pressure. Not surprisingly, there is no enhanced expression of caveolin-1 in SMCs. However, caveolin-1 and eNOS dysfunction lead to SMC proliferation, medial hypertrophy and loss of endothelial-dependent vascular relaxation. Removal of hypoxia results in the disruption of caveolin-1/eNOS tight complex leading to reversal of PH. Slowly, the pulmonary artery pressure and medial hypertrophy return to normal as seen in experimental animals and in people returning to sea level from high altitude. Hypoxia-induced PH is reversible. However, associated inflammation/shear stress in hypoxia-induced PH, resulting in EC disruption, would lead to irreversible PH.

In conclusion, EC integrity and caveolin-1 function are important factors that determine reversible vs. irreversible PH.

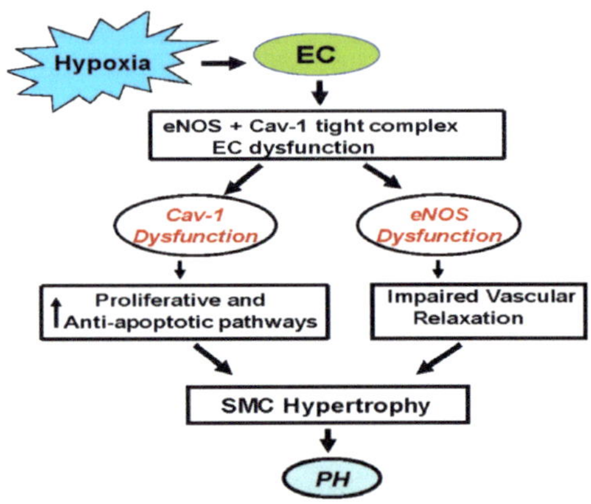

Figure 2.
This figure shows the effect of hypoxia on EC leading to eNOS/caveolin-1 complex formation, endothelial dysfunction and subsequent medial hypertrophy and PH. EC = endothelial cells, Cav-1 = caveolin-1, eNOS = endothelial nitric oxide synthase, SMC = smooth muscle cells, PH = pulmonary hypertension.

Acknowledgements

This work is in part supported by Cardiovascular Medical Research and Education Fund.

Author details

Rajamma Mathew
Department of Pediatrics, Section of Pediatric Cardiology, New York Medical College, Valhalla, NY, USA

*Address all correspondence to: rajamma_mathew@NYMC.edu

References

[1] Simonneau G, Gatzoulis MA, Adatia I, Celermajer D, Denton C, Ghofrani A, et al. Updated clinical classification of pulmonary hypertension. Journal of the American College of Cardiology. 2013;**62**(25 Suppl):D34-D41. DOI: 10.1016/j.jacc.2013.10.029

[2] Best DH, Sumner KL, Smith BP, Damjanovich-Colmenares K, Nakayama I, Brown LM, et al. EIF2AK4 mutations in patients diagnosed with pulmonary arterial hypertension. Chest. 2017;**151**:821-828. DOI: 10.1016/j.chest.2016.11.014

[3] Simonneau G, Montani D, Celermajer DS, Denton CP, Gatzoulis MA, Krowka M, et al. Haemodynamic definitions and updated clinical classification of pulmonary hypertension. European Respiratory Journal. 2019;**53**(1). DOI: 10.1183/13993003.01913-2018

[4] Kovacs G, Berghold A, Scheidl S, Olschewski H. Pulmonary arterial pressure during rest and exercise in healthy subjects: A systematic review. The European Respiratory Journal. 2009;**34**:888-894. DOI: 10.1183/09031936.00145608

[5] Hoeper MM, Humbert M, Souza R, Idrees M, Kawut SM, Sliwa-Hahnle K, et al. A global view of pulmonary hypertension. The Lancet Respiratory Medicine. 2016;**4**:306-322. DOI: 10.1016/S2213-2600(15)00543-3

[6] Thenappan T, Shah SJ, Rich S, Tian L, Archer SL, Gomberg-Maitland M. Survival in pulmonary arterial hypertension: A reappraisal of the NIH risk stratification equation. The European Respiratory Journal. 2010;**35**:1079-1087. DOI: 10.1183/09031936.00072709

[7] Pogoriler JE, Rich S, Archer SL, Husain AN. Persistence of complex vascular lesions despite prolonged prostacyclin therapy of pulmonary arterial hypertension. Histopathology. 2012;**61**:597-609. DOI: 10.1111/j.1365-2559.2012.04246.x

[8] Strange G, Gabbay E, Kermeen F, Williams T, Carrington M, Stewart S, et al. Time from symptoms to definitive diagnosis of idiopathic pulmonary arterial hypertension: The delay study. Pulmonary Circulation. 2013;**3**:89-94. DOI: 10.4103/2045-8932.109919

[9] Huang J, Wolk JH, Gewitz MH, Mathew R. Progressive endothelial cell damage in an inflammatory model of pulmonary hypertension. Experimental Lung Research. 2010;**36**:57-66. DOI: 10.3109/01902140903104793

[10] Mathew R. Pulmonary hypertension management challenges in pediatric age group. Annals of Vascular Medicine and Research. 2017;**4**(3):1057

[11] Muensterer O, Abellar R, Otterburn D, Mathew R. Pulmonary agenesis and associated pulmonary hypertension: A case report and review on variability, therapy, and outcome. European Journal of Pediatric Surgery Reports. 2015;**3**:33-39. DOI: 10.1055/s-0034-1395986

[12] van Loon RL, Roofthooft MT, Hillege HL, ten Harkel AD, van Osch-Gevers M, Delhass T, et al. Pediatric pulmonary hypertension in Netherlands: Epidemiology and characterization during period 1991 to 2005. Circulation. 2011;**124**:1755-1764. DOI: 10.1161/CIRCULATIONAHA.110.969584

[13] Naumburg E, Söderström L, Huber D, Axelsson I. Risk factors for pulmonary arterial hypertension in children and young adults. Pediatric Pulmonology. 2017;**52**:636-641. DOI: 10.1002/ppul.23633

[14] Chida A, Shintani M, Yagi H, Fujiwara M, Kojima Y, Sato H, et al. Outcomes of childhood pulmonary arterial hypertension in BMPR2 and ALK1 mutation carriers. The American Journal of Cardiology. 2012;**110**:586-593. DOI: 10.1016/j.amjcard.2012.04.035

[15] Galambos C, Mullen MP, Shieh JT, Schwerk N, Kielt MJ, Ullmann N, et al. Phenotype characterisation of *TBX4* mutation and deletion carriers with neonatal and pediatric pulmonary hypertension. European Respiratory Journal. 2019;**54**(2):1801965. DOI: 10.1183/13993003.01965-2018

[16] Rabinovitch M, Keane JF, Norwood WI, Castaneda AR, Reid L. Vascular structure in lung tissue obtained at biopsy correlated with pulmonary hemodynamic findings after repair of congenital heart defects. Circulation. 1984;**69**:655-667. DOI: 10.1161/01.cir.69.4.655

[17] Yamaki S, Wagenvoort CA. Comparison of primary plexogenic arteriopathy in adults and children. A morphometric study in 40 patients. British Heart Journal. 1985;**54**:428-434. DOI: 10.1136/hrt.54.4.428

[18] Lee SD, Shroyer KR, Markham NE, Cool CD, Voelkel NF, Tuder RM. Monoclonal endothelial cell proliferation is present in primary but not secondary pulmonary hypertension. The Journal of Clinical Investigation. 1998;**101**:927-934. DOI: 10.1172/JCI1910

[19] Ranchoux B, Harvey LD, Ayon RJ, Babicheva A, Bonnet S, Chan SY, et al. Endothelial dysfunction in pulmonary arterial hypertension: An evolving landscape (2017 Grover conference series). Pulmonary Circulation. 2018;**8**:2045893217752912. DOI: 10.1177/2045893217752912

[20] Humbert M, Morrell NW, Archer SL, Stenmark KR, MacLean MR, Lang IM, et al. Cellular and molecular pathobiology of pulmonary arterial hypertension. Journal of the American College of Cardiology. 2004;**43**(12 Suppl S):13S-24S. DOI: 10.1016/j.jacc.2004.02.029

[21] Mathew R. Inflammation and pulmonary hypertension. Cardiology in Review. 2010;**18**:67-72. DOI: 10.1097/CRD.0b013e3181cd612f

[22] Balabanian K, Foussat A, Dorfmüller P, Durand-Gasselin I, Capel F, Bouchet-Delbos L, et al. CX (3) C chemokine fractalkine in pulmonary arterial hypertension. American Journal of Respiratory and Critical Care Medicine. 2002;**165**:1419-1425. DOI: 10.1164/rccm.2106007

[23] Dorfmüller P, Zarka V, Durand-Gasselin I, Monti G, Balabanian K, Garcia G, et al. Chemokine RANTES in severe pulmonary arterial hypertension. American Journal of Respiratory and Critical Care Medicine. 2002;**165**:534-539. DOI: 10.1164/ajrccm.165.4.2012112

[24] Nie X, Tan J, Dai Y, Liu Y, Zou J, Sun J, et al. CCL5 deficiency rescues pulmonary vascular dysfunction, and reverses pulmonary hypertension via caveolin-1-dependent BMPR2 activation. Journal of Molecular and Cellular Cardiology. 2018;**116**:41-56. DOI: 10.1016/j.yjmcc.2018.01.016

[25] Tuder RM, Groves B, Badesch DB, Voelkel NF. Exuberant endothelial cell growth and elements of inflammation are present in plexiform lesions of pulmonary hypertension. The American Journal of Pathology. 1994;**144**:275-285

[26] Stacher E, Graham BB, Hunt JM, Gandjeva A, Groshong SD, McLaughlin VV, et al. Modern age pathology of pulmonary arterial hypertension. American Journal of Respiratory and Critical Care Medicine. 2012;**186**:261-272. DOI: 10.1164/rccm.201201-0164OC

[27] Humbert M, Monti G, Brenot F, Sitbon O, Portier A, Grangeot-Keros L, et al. Increased interleukin-1 and interleukin-6 serum concentrations in severe primary pulmonary hypertension. American Journal of Respiratory and Critical Care Medicine. 1995;**151**:1628-q631. DOI: 10.1164/ajrccm.151.5.7735624

[28] Bhargava A, Kumar A, Yuan N, Gewitz MH, Mathew R. Monocrotaline induces interleukin-6 mRNA expression in rat lungs. Heart Disease. 1999;**1**:126-132

[29] Schermuly RT, Ghofrani HA, Wilkins MR, Grimminger F. Mechanisms of disease: Pulmonary arterial hypertension. Nature Reviews. Cardiology. 2011;**8**:443-455. DOI: 10.1038/nrcardio.2011.87

[30] Xu W, Erzurum SC. Endothelial cell energy metabolism, proliferation, and apoptosis in pulmonary hypertension. Comprehensive Physiology. 2011;**1**:357-372. DOI: 10.1002/cphy.c090005

[31] Mathew R, Huang J, Shah M, Patel K, Gewitz M, Sehgal PB. Disruption of endothelial-cell caveolin-1alpha/raft scaffolding during development of monocrotaline-induced pulmonary hypertension. Circulation. 2004;**110**:1499-1506. DOI: 10.1161/01.CIR.0000141576.39579.23

[32] Masri FA, Xu W, Comhair SA, Asosingh K, Koo M, Vasanji A, et al. Hyperproliferative apoptosis-resistant endothelial cells in idiopathic pulmonary arterial hypertension. American Journal of Physiology. Lung Cellular and Molecular Physiology. 2007;**293**:L548-L554. DOI: 10.1152/ajplung.00428.2006

[33] Shibata R, Kai H, Seki Y, Kato S, Wada Y, Hanakawa Y, et al. Inhibition of STAT3 prevents neointima formation by inhibiting proliferation and promoting apoptosis of neointimal smooth muscle cells. Human Gene Therapy. 2003;**14**:601-610. DOI: 10.1089/104303403321618128

[34] Soon E, Crosby A, Southwood M, Yang P, Tajsic T, Toshner M, et al. Bone morphogenetic protein receptor type II deficiency and increased inflammatory cytokine production. A gateway to pulmonary arterial hypertension. American Journal of Respiratory and Critical Care Medicine. 2015;**192**:859-872. DOI: 10.1164/rccm.201408-1509OC

[35] Brock M, Trenkmann M, Gay RE, Michel BA, Gay S, Fischler M, et al. Interleukin-6 modulates the expression of the bone morphogenic protein receptor type II through a novel STAT3-microRNA cluster 17/92 pathway. Circulation Research. 2009;**104**:1184-1191. DOI: 10.1161/CIRCRESAHA.109.197491

[36] Atkinson C, Stewart S, Upton PD, Machado R, Thomson JR, Trembath RC, et al. Primary pulmonary hypertension is associated with reduced pulmonary vascular expression of type II bone morphogenetic protein receptor. Circulation. 2002;**105**:1672-1678. DOI: 10.1161/01.cir.0000012754.72951.3d

[37] Murakami K, Mathew R, Huang J, Farahani R, Peng H, Olson SC, et al. Smurf1 ubiquitin ligase causes downregulation of BMP receptors and is induced in monocrotaline and hypoxia models of pulmonary arterial hypertension. Experimental Biology and Medicine. 2010;**235**:805-813. DOI: 10.1258/ebm.2010.009383

[38] Rothman AM, Arnold ND, Pickworth JA, Iremonger J, Ciuclan L, Allen RM, et al. MicroRNA-140-5p and SMURF1 regulate pulmonary arterial hypertension. Journal of Clinical Sciences. 2016;**126**:2495-2508. DOI: 10.1172/JCI83361

[39] Nickel NP, Spiekerkoetter E, Gu M, Li CG, Li H, Kaschwich M, et al. Elafin

reverses pulmonary hypertension via caveolin-1-dependent bone morphogenetic protein signaling. American Journal of Respiratory and Critical Care Medicine. 2015;**191**(11):1273-1286. DOI: 10.1164/rccm.201412-2291OC

[40] Dabral S, Tian X, Kojonazarov B, Savai R, Ghofrani HA, Weissmann N, et al. Notch1 signalling regulates endothelial proliferation and apoptosis in pulmonary arterial hypertension. The European Respiratory Journal. 2016;**48**:1137-1149. DOI: 10.1183/13993003.00773-2015

[41] Zou J, Li P, Lu F, Liu N, Dai J, Ye J, et al. Notch1 is required for hypoxia-induced proliferation, invasion and chemoresistance of T-cell acute lymphoblastic leukemia cells. Journal of Hematology & Oncology. 2013;**6**:3. DOI: 10.1186/1756-8722-6-3

[42] Takeshita K, Satoh M, Ii M, Silver M, Limbourg FP, Mukai Y, et al. Critical role of endothelial Notch1 signaling in postnatal angiogenesis. Circulation Research. 2007;**100**:70-78. DOI: 10.1161/01.RES.0000254788.47304.6e

[43] Mack JJ, Iruela-Arispe ML. NOTCH regulation of the endothelial cell phenotype. Current Opinion in Hematology. 2018;**25**:212-218. DOI: 10.1097/MOH.0000000000000425

[44] Mack JJ, Mosqueiro TS, Archer BJ, Jones WM, Sunshine H, Faas GC, et al. NOTCH1 is a mechanosensor in adult arteries. Nature Communications. 2017;**8**:1620. DOI: 10.1038/s41467-017-01741-8

[45] Serra H, Chivite I, Angulo-Urarte A, Soler A, Sutherland JD, Arruabarrena-Aristorena A, et al. PTEN mediates notch-dependent stalk cell arrest in angiogenesis. Nature Communications. 2015;**6**:7935. DOI: 10.1038/ncomms8935

[46] Huang J, Frid M, Gewitz MH, Fallon JT, Brown D, Krafsur G, et al. Hypoxia-induced pulmonary hypertension and chronic lung disease: Caveolin-1 dysfunction an important underlying feature. Pulmonary Circulation. 2019;**9**(1):2045894019837876. DOI: 10.1177/2045894019837876

[47] Xia H, Khalil W, Kahm J, Jessurun J, Kleidon J, Henke CA. Pathologic caveolin-1 regulation of PTEN in idiopathic pulmonary fibrosis. The American Journal of Pathology. 2010;**176**:2626-2637. DOI: 10.2353/ajpath.2010.091117

[48] Sun S, Steinberg BM. PTEN is a negative regulator of STAT3 activation in human papillomavirus-infected cells. The Journal of General Virology. 2002;**83**:1651-1658. DOI: 10.1099/0022-1317-83-7-1651

[49] Mathew R. Pulmonary hypertension: Endothelial cell function. In: Sulica R, Preston I, editors. Pulmonary Hypertension: From Bench Research to Clinical Challenge. Croatia: IntechOpen; 2011. pp. 1-24. ISBN: 978-953-307-835-9

[50] Dorland YL, Huveneers S. Cell-cell junctional mechanotransduction in endothelial remodeling. Cellular and Molecular Life Sciences. 2017;**74**:279-292. DOI: 10.1007/s00018-016-2325-8

[51] Palade GE. Fine structure of blood capillaries. Journal of Applied Physiology. 1953;**24**:1424

[52] Yamada E. The fine structure of the gall bladder epithelium of the mouse. The Journal of Biophysical and Biochemical Cytology. 1955;**1**:445-458. DOI: 10.1083/jcb.1.5.445

[53] Couet J, Li S, Okamoto T, Ikezu T, Lisanti MP. Identification of peptide and protein ligands for the caveolin-scaffolding domain. Implications

for the interaction of caveolin with caveolae-associated proteins. The Journal of Biological Chemistry. 1997;**272**(10):6525-6533. DOI: 10.1074/jbc.272.10.6525

[54] Parton RG, del Pozo MA. Caveolae as plasma membrane sensors, protectors and organizers. Nature Reviews. Molecular Cell Biology. 2013;**14**:98-112. DOI: 10.1038/nrm3512

[55] Sinha B, Köster D, Ruez R, Gonnord P, Bastiani M, Abankwa D, et al. Cells respond to mechanical stress by rapid disassembly of caveolae. Cell. 2011;**144**:402-413. DOI: 10.1016/j.cell.2010.12.031

[56] Frank PG, Woodman SE, Park DS, Lisanti MP. Caveolin, caveolae, and endothelial cell function. Arteriosclerosis, Thrombosis, and Vascular Biology. 2003;**23**:1161-1168. DOI: 10.1161/01.ATV.0000070546.16946.3A

[57] Shaul PW, Anderson RG. Role of plasmalemmal caveolae in signal transduction. The American Journal of Physiology. 1998;**275**:L843-L851. DOI: 10.1152/ajplung.1998.275.5.L843

[58] Le PU, Guay G, Altschuler Y, Nabi IR. Caveolin-1 is a negative regulator of caveolae-mediated endocytosis to the endoplasmic reticulum. The Journal of Biological Chemistry. 2002;**277**:3371-3379. DOI: 10.1074/jbc.M111240200

[59] Parton RG, Simons K. The multiple faces of caveolae. Nature Reviews. Molecular Cell Biology. 2007;**8**:185-194. DOI: 10.1038/nrm2122

[60] Ariotti N, Rae J, Leneva N, Ferguson C, Loo D, Okano S, et al. Molecular characterization of caveolin-induced membrane curvature. The Journal of Biological Chemistry. 2015;**290**:24875-24890. DOI: 10.1074/jbc.M115.644336

[61] Okamoto T, Schlegel A, Scherer PE, Lisanti MP. Caveolins, a family of scaffolding proteins for organizing "preassembled signaling complexes" at the plasma membrane. The Journal of Biological Chemistry. 1998;**273**:5419-5422. DOI: 10.1074/jbc.273.10.5419

[62] Mathew R. PDGF receptor blocker for pulmonary hypertension: A new agent in therapeutic arsenal. Expert Opinion on Investigational Drugs. 2012;**21**:139-142. DOI: 10.1517/13543784.2012.650861

[63] Jasmin JF, Mercier I, Sotgia F, Lisanti MP. SOCS proteins and caveolin-1 as negative regulators of endocrine signaling. Trends in Endocrinology and Metabolism. 2006;**17**:150-158. DOI: 10.1016/j.tem.2006.03.007

[64] Fujimoto T, Kogo H, Nomura R, Une T. Isoforms of caveolin-1 and caveolar structure. Journal of Cell Science. 2000;**113**(Pt 19):3509-3517

[65] Parolini I, Sargiacomo M, Galbiati F, Rizzo G, Grignani F, Engelman JA, et al. Expression of caveolin-1 is required for the transport of caveolin-2 to the plasma membrane. Retention of caveolin-2 at the level of the golgi complex. The Journal of Biological Chemistry. 1999;**274**:25718-25725. DOI: 10.1074/jbc.274.36.25718

[66] Xie L, Frank PG, Lisanti MP, Sowa G. Endothelial cells isolated from caveolin-2 knockout mice display higher proliferation rate and cell cycle progression relative to their wild-type counterparts. American Journal of Physiology. Cell Physiology. 2010;**298**:C693-C701. DOI: 10.1152/ajpcell.00401.2009

[67] Razani B, Wang XB, Engelman JA, Battista M, Lagaud G, Zhang XL, et al. Caveolin-2-deficient mice show evidence of severe pulmonary dysfunction without

disruption of caveolae. Molecular and Cellular Biology. 2002;**22**:2329-2344. DOI: 10.1128/MCB.22.7.2329-2344.2002

[68] Liu L, Pilch PF. A critical role of cavin (polymerase I and transcript release factor) in caveolae formation and organization. The Journal of Biological Chemistry. 2008;**283**:4314-4322. DOI: 10.1074/jbc.M707890200

[69] Hill MM, Bastiani M, Luetterforst R, Kirkham M, Kirkham A, Nixon SJ, et al. PTRF-Cavin, a conserved cytoplasmic protein required for caveola formation and function. Cell. 2008;**132**:113-124. DOI: 10.1016/j.cell.2007.11.042

[70] Dávalos A, Fernández-Hernando C, Sowa G, Derakhshan B, Lin MI, Lee JY, et al. Quantitative proteomics of caveolin-1-regulated proteins: Characterization of polymerase 1 and transcript release factor/CAVIN-1 in endothelial cells. Molecular & Cellular Proteomics. 2010;**9**:2109-2124. DOI: 10.1074/mcp.M110.001289

[71] Zhou LJ, Chen XY, Liu SP, Zhang LL, Xu YN, Mu PW, et al. Downregulation of Cavin-1 expression via increasing caveolin-1 degradation prompts the proliferation and migration of vascular smooth muscle cells in balloon injury-induced neointimal hyperplasia. Journal of American Heart Association. 2017;**6**(8). DOI: 10.1161/JAHA.117.005754

[72] Swärd K, Sadegh MK, Mori M, Erjefält JS, Rippe C. Elevated pulmonary arterial pressure and altered expression of Ddah1 and Arg1 in mice lacking cavin-1/PTRF. Physiological Reports. 2013;**1**(1):e00008. DOI: 10.1002/PHY2.8

[73] Liu L, Brown D, McKee M, Lebrasseur NK, Yang D, Albrecht KH, et al. Deletion of Cavin/PTRF causes global loss of caveolae, dyslipidemia, and glucose intolerance. Cell Metabolism. 2008;**8**:310-317. DOI: 10.1016/j.cmet.2008.07.008

[74] Hansen CG, Howard G, Nichols BJ. Pacsin 2 is recruited to caveolae and functions in caveolar biogenesis. Journal of Cell Science. 2011;**124**:2777-2785. DOI: 10.1242/jcs.084319

[75] Hoernke M, Mohan J, Larsson E, Blomberg J, Kahra D, Westenhoff S, et al. EHD2 restrains dynamics of caveolae by an ATP-dependent, membrane-bound, open conformation. Proceedings of the National Academy of Sciences. 2017;**114**:E4360-E4369. DOI: 10.1073/pnas.1614066114

[76] Lamaze C, Tardif N, Dewulf M, Vassilopoulos S, Blouin CM. The caveolae dress code: Structure and signaling. Current Opinion in Cell Biology. 2017;**47**:117-125. DOI: 10.1016/j.ceb.2017.02.014

[77] Drab M, Verkade P, Elger M, Kasper M, Lohn M, Lauterbach B, et al. Loss of caveolae, vascular dysfunction, and pulmonary defects in caveolin-1 gene-disrupted mice. Science. 2001;**293**(5539):2449-2452. DOI: 10.1126/science.1062688

[78] Murata T, Lin MI, Huang Y, Yu J, Bauer PM, Giordano FJ, et al. Re-expression of caveolin-1 in endothelium rescues the vascular, cardiac, and pulmonary defects in global caveolin-1 knockout mice. The Journal of Experimental Medicine. 2007;**204**:2373-2382. DOI: 10.1084/jem.20062340

[79] Codrici E, Albulescu L, Popescu ID, Mihai S, Enciu AM, Albulescu R, et al. Caveolin-1-knockout mouse as a model of inflammatory diseases. Journal of Immunology Research. 2018;**2018**:2498576. DOI: 10.1155/2018/2498576. eCollection 2018

[80] Oliveira SDS, Castellon M, Chen J, Bonini MG, Gu X, Elliott MH, et al. Inflammation-induced caveolin-1 and BMPRII depletion promotes

endothelial dysfunction and TGF-β-driven pulmonary vascular remodeling. American Journal of Physiology. Lung Cellular and Molecular Physiology. 2017;**312**:L760-L771. DOI: 10.1152/ajplung.00484.2016

[81] Cho JG, Lee A, Chang W, Lee MS, Kim J. Endothelial to mesenchymal transition represents a key link in the interaction between inflammation and endothelial dysfunction. Frontiers in Immunology. 2018;**9**:294. DOI: 10.3389/fimmu.2018.00294 eCollection 2018

[82] Shiroto T, Romero N, Sugiyama T, Sartoretto JL, Kalwa H, Yan Z, et al. Caveolin-1 is a critical determinant of autophagy, metabolic switching, and oxidative stress in vascular endothelium. PLoS One. 2014;**9**:e87871. DOI: 10.1371/journal.pone.0087871. eCollection 2014

[83] Michel JB, Feron O, Sacks D, Michel T. Reciprocal regulation of endothelial nitric-oxide synthase by Ca^{2+}–calmodulin and caveolin. The Journal of Biological Chemistry. 1997;**272**:15583-15586. DOI: 10.1074/jbc.272.25.15583

[84] Bernatchez PN, Bauer PM, Yu J, Prendergast JS, He P, Sessa WC. Dissecting the molecular control of endothelial NO synthase by caveolin-1 using cell-permeable peptides. Proceedings of the National Academy of Sciences. 2005;**102**:761-7666. DOI: 10.1073/pnas.0407224102

[85] García-Cardeña G, Martasek P, Masters BS, Skidd PM, Couet J, Li S, et al. Dissecting the interaction between nitric oxide synthase (NOS) and caveolin. Functional significance of the NOS caveolin binding domain in vivo. The Journal of Biological Chemistry. 1997;**272**:25437-25440. DOI: 10.1074/jbc.272.41.25437

[86] Rizzo V, McIntosh DP, Oh P, Schnitzer JE. In situ flow activates endothelial nitric oxide synthase in luminal caveolae of endothelium with rapid caveolin dissociation and calmodulin association. The Journal of Biological Chemistry. 1998;**273**:34724-34729. DOI: 10.1074/jbc.273.52.34724

[87] Chidlow JH Jr, Sessa WC. Caveolae, caveolins, and cavins: Complex control of cellular signalling and inflammation. Cardiovascular Research. 2010;**86**:219-225. DOI: 10.1093/cvr/cvq075

[88] Oliveira SDS, Minshall RD. Caveolin and endothelial NO signaling. Current Topics in Membranes. 2018;**82**:257-279. DOI: 10.1016/bs.ctm.2018.09.004

[89] Tian J, Hou Y, Lu Q, Wiseman DA, Vasconcelos Fonsesca F, Elms S, et al. A novel role for caveolin-1 in regulating endothelial nitric oxide synthase activation in response to H_2O_2 and shear stress. Free Radical Biology & Medicine. 2010;**49**:159-170. DOI: 10.1016/j.freeradbiomed.2010.03.023

[90] Sonveaux P, Martinive P, DeWever J, Batova Z, Daneau G, Pelat M, et al. Caveolin-1 expression is critical for vascular endothelial growth factor-induced ischemic hindlimb collateralization and nitric oxide-mediated angiogenesis. Circulation Research. 2004;**95**:154-161. DOI: 10.1161/01.RES.0000136344.27825.72

[91] Morais C, Ebrahem Q, Anand-Apte B, Parat MO. Altered angiogenesis in caveolin-1 gene-deficient mice is restored by ablation of endothelial nitric oxide synthase. The American Journal of Pathology. 2012;**180**:1702-1714. DOI: 10.1016/j.ajpath.2011.12.018

[92] Rath G, Dessy C, Feron O. Caveolae, caveolin and control of vascular tone: Nitric oxide (NO) and endothelium derived hyperpolarizing factor (EDHF) regulation. Journal of Physiology and Pharmacology. 2009;**60**(Suppl. 4):105-109

[93] Goedicke-Fritz S, Kaistha A, Kacik M, Markert S, Hofmeister A,

Busch C, et al. Evidence for functional and dynamic microcompartmentation of Cav-1/TRPV4/K(Ca) in caveolae of endothelial cells. European Journal of Cell Biology. 2015;**94**:391-400. DOI: 10.1016/j.ejcb.2015.06.002

[94] Saliez J, Bouzin C, Rath G, Ghisdal P, Desjardins F, Rezzani R, et al. Role of caveolar compartmentation in endothelium-derived hyperpolarizing factor-mediated relaxation: Ca^{2+} signals and gap junction function are regulated by caveolin in endothelial cells. Circulation. 2008;**117**:1065-1074. DOI: 10.1161/CIRCULATIONAHA.107.731679

[95] Spisni E, Griffoni C, Santi S, Riccio M, Marulli R, Bartolini G, et al. Colocalization prostacyclin (PGI2) synthase—Caveolin-1 in endothelial cells and new roles for PGI2 in angiogenesis. Experimental Cell Research. 2001;**266**:31-43. DOI: 10.1006/excr.2001.5198

[96] Mathew R. Pathogenesis of pulmonary hypertension: A case for caveolin-1 and cell membrane integrity. American Journal of Physiology. Heart and Circulatory Physiology. 2014;**306**:H15-H25. DOI: 10.1152/ajpheart.00266.2013

[97] Zeng Y. Endothelial glycocalyx as a critical signalling platform integrating the extracellular haemodynamic forces and chemical signalling. Journal of Cellular and Molecular Medicine. 2017;**21**:1457-1462. DOI: 10.1111/jcmm.13081

[98] Harding IC, Mitra R, Mensah SA, Herman IM, Ebong EE. Pro-atherosclerotic disturbed flow disrupts caveolin-1 expression, localization, and function via glycocalyx degradation. Journal of Translational Medicine. 2018;**16**:364. DOI: 10.1186/s12967-018-1721-2

[99] Guo J, Yang ZC, Liu Y. Attenuating pulmonary hypertension by protecting the integrity of glycocalyx in rats model of pulmonary artery hypertension. Inflammation. 2019. DOI: 10.1007/s10753-019-01055-5

[100] Gavard J. Endothelial permeability and VE-cadherin: A wacky comradeship. Cell Adhesion & Migration. 2014;**8**:158-164. DOI: 10.4161/cam.29026

[101] Kronstein R, Seebach J, Grossklaus S, Minten C, Engelhardt B, Drab M, et al. Caveolin-1 opens endothelial cell junctions by targeting catenins. Cardiovascular Research. 2012;**93**:130-140. DOI: 10.1093/cvr/cvr256

[102] Caveda L, Martin-Padura I, Navarro P, Breviario F, Corada M, Gulino D, et al. Inhibition of cultured cell growth by vascular endothelial cadherin (cadherin-5/VE-cadherin). The Journal of Clinical Investigation. 1996;**98**:886-893. DOI: 10.1172/JCI118870

[103] Song L, Ge S, Pachter JS. Caveolin-1 regulates expression of junction-associated proteins in brain microvascular endothelial cells. Blood. 2007;**109**:1515-1523. DOI: 10.1182/blood-2006-07-034009

[104] Dejana E, Giampietro C. Vascular endothelial-cadherin and vascular stability. Current Opinion in Hematology. 2012;**9**:218-223. DOI: 10.1097/MOH.0b013e3283523e1c

[105] Vestweber D. VE-cadherin: The major endothelial adhesion molecule controlling cellular junctions and blood vessel formation. Arteriosclerosis, Thrombosis, and Vascular Biology. 2008;**28**:223-232. DOI: 10.1161/ATVBAHA.107.158014

[106] Le Guelte A, Dwyer J, Gavard J. Jumping the barrier: VE-cadherin, VEGF and other angiogenic modifiers in cancer. Biology of the Cell. 2011;**103**:593-605. DOI: 10.1042/BC20110069

[107] Nikitopoulou I, Orfanos SE, Kotanidou A, Maltabe V, Manitsopoulos N, Karras P, et al. Vascular endothelial-cadherin downregulation as a feature of endothelial transdifferentiation in monocrotaline-induced pulmonary hypertension. American Journal of Physiology. Lung Cellular and Molecular Physiology. 2016;**311**:L352-L363. DOI: 10.1152/ajplung.00156.2014

[108] Privratsky JR, Newman PJ. PECAM-1: Regulator of endothelial junctional integrity. Cell and Tissue Research. 2014;**355**:607-619. DOI: 10.1007/s00441-013-1779-3

[109] Burton VJ, Ciuclan LI, Holmes AM, Rodman DM, Walker C, Budd DC. Bone morphogenetic protein receptor II regulates pulmonary artery endothelial cell barrier function. Blood. 2011;**117**:333-341. DOI: 10.1182/blood-2010-05-285973

[110] Mathew R. Cell-specific dual role of caveolin-1 in pulmonary hypertension. Pulmonary Medicine. 2011;**2011**:573432. DOI: 10.1155/2011/573432

[111] Kim J, Hwangbo C, Hu X, Kang Y, Papangeli I, Mehrotra D, et al. Restoration of impaired endothelial myocyte enhancer factor 2 function rescues pulmonary arterial hypertension. Circulation. 2015;**131**:190-199. DOI: 10.1161/CIRCULATIONAHA.114.013339

[112] Huertas A, Tu L, Thuillet R, Le Hiress M, Phan C, Ricard N, et al. Leptin signalling system as a target for pulmonary arterial hypertension therapy. The European Respiratory Journal. 2015;**45**:1066-1080. DOI: 10.1183/09031936.00193014

[113] Tu L, Dewachter L, Gore B, Fadel E, Dartevelle P, Simonneau G, et al. Autocrine fibroblast growth factor-2 signaling contributes to altered endothelial phenotype in pulmonary hypertension. American Journal of Respiratory Cell and Molecular Biology. 2011;**45**:311-322. DOI: 10.1165/rcmb.2010-0317OC

[114] Le Hiress M, Tu L, Ricard N, Phan C, Thuillet R, Fadel E, et al. Proinflammatory signature of the dysfunctional endothelium in pulmonary hypertension. Role of the macrophage migration inhibitory factor/CD74 complex. American Journal of Respiratory and Critical Care Medicine. 2015;**192**(8):983-997. DOI: 10.1164/rccm.201402-0322OC

[115] Jasmin JF, Mercier I, Hnasko R, Cheung MW, Tanowitz HB, Dupuis J, et al. Lung remodeling and pulmonary hypertension after myocardial infarction: Pathogenic role of reduced caveolin expression. Cardiovascular Research. 2004;**63**:747-755. DOI: 10.1016/j.cardiores.2004.05.018

[116] Achcar RO, Demura Y, Rai PR, Taraseviciene-Stewart L, Kasper M, Voelkel NF, et al. Loss of caveolin and heme oxygenase expression in severe pulmonary hypertension. Chest. 2006;**129**:696-705. DOI: 10.1378/chest.129.3.696

[117] Huang J, Wolk JH, Gewitz MH, Mathew R. Caveolin-1 expression during the progression of pulmonary hypertension. Experimental Biology and Medicine. 2012;**237**:956-965. DOI: 10.1258/ebm.2012.011382

[118] Mathew R, Guzowski DE, Gloster ES. Effect of verapamil on monocrotaline-induced pulmonary artery hypertension and endothelial cell dysfunction in rats. Experimental Lung Research. 1990;**16**:627-644

[119] Huang J, Kaminski PM, Edwards JG, Yeh A, Wolin MS, Frishman WH, et al. Pyrrolidine dithiocarbamate restores endothelial cell membrane integrity and attenuates monocrotaline-induced

pulmonary artery hypertension. American Journal of Physiology. Lung Cellular and Molecular Physiology. 2008;**294**:L1250-L1259. DOI: 10.1152/ajplung.00069.2007

[120] Jasmin JF, Mercier I, Dupuis J, Tanowitz HB, Lisanti MP. Short-term administration of a cell-permeable caveolin-1 peptide prevents the development of monocrotaline-induced pulmonary hypertension and right ventricular hypertrophy. Circulation. 2006;**114**(9):912-920. DOI: 10.1161/CIRCULATIONAHA.106.634709

[121] Mathew R. Possible mechanism of neointima formation in pulmonary arterial hypertension. Blood, Heart and Circulation. 2018;**2**:1-5. DOI: 10.15761/BHC1000145

[122] Huang J, Wolk JH, Gewitz MH, Loyd JE, West J, Austin ED, et al. Enhanced caveolin-1 expression in smooth muscle cells: Possible prelude to neointima formation. World Journal of Cardiology. 2015;**7**:671-684. DOI: 10.4330/wjc.v7.i10.671

[123] Dereddy N, Huang J, Erb M, Guzel S, Wolk JH, Sett SS, et al. Associated inflammation or increased flow-mediated shear stress, but not pressure alone, disrupts endothelial caveolin-1 in infants with pulmonary hypertension. Pulmonary Circulation. 2012;**2**:492-500. DOI: 10.4103/2045-8932.105038

[124] Mathew R, Huang J, Katta US, Krishnan U, Sandoval C, Gewitz MH. Immunosuppressant-inducedendothelial damage and pulmonary arterial hypertension. Journal of Pediatric Hematology/Oncology. 2011;**33**:55-58. DOI: 10.1097/MPH.0b013e3181ec0ede

[125] Patel HH, Zhang S, Murray F, Suda RY, Head BP, Yokoyama U, et al. Increased smooth muscle cell expression of caveolin-1 and caveolae contribute to the pathophysiology of idiopathic pulmonary arterial hypertension. The FASEB Journal. 2007;**21**(11):2970-2979. DOI: 10.1096/fj.07-8424com

[126] Huang J, Mathew R. Loss of cavin1 and expression of p-caveolin-1 in pulmonary hypertension: Possible role in neointima formation. World Journal of Hypertension. 2019;**9**:17-29. DOI: 10.5494/wjh.v9.i2.17

[127] Ortiz R, Díaz J, Díaz N, Lobos-Gonzalez L, Cárdenas A, Contreras P, et al. Extracellular matrix-specific Caveolin-1 phosphorylation on tyrosine 14 is linked to augmented melanoma metastasis but not tumorigenesis. Oncotarget. 2016;7:40571-40593. DOI: 10.18632/oncotarget.9738

[128] Joshi B, Strugnell SS, Goetz JG, Kojic LD, Cox ME, Griffith OL, et al. Phosphorylated caveolin-1 regulates rho/ROCK-dependent focal adhesion dynamics and tumor cell migration and invasion. Cancer Research. 2008;**68**:8210-8220. DOI: 10.1158/0008-5472.CAN-08-0343

[129] Sakao S, Tatsumi K, Voelkel NF. Reversible or irreversible remodeling in pulmonary arterial hypertension. American Journal of Respiratory Cell and Molecular Biology. 2010;**43**:629-634. DOI: 10.1165/rcmb.2009-0389TR

[130] Okada K, Tanaka Y, Bernstein M, Zhang W, Patterson GA, Botney MD. Pulmonary hemodynamics modify the rat pulmonary artery response to injury. A neointimal model of pulmonary hypertension. The American Journal of Pathology. 1997;**151**:1019-1025

[131] Tanaka Y, Schuster DP, Davis EC, Patterson GA, Botney MD. The role of vascular injury and hemodynamics in rat pulmonary artery remodeling. The Journal of Clinical Investigation. 1996;**98**:434-442

[132] Dammann JF Jr, McEachen JA, Thompson WM Jr, Smith R, Muller

WH Jr. The regression of pulmonary vascular disease after the creation of pulmonary stenosis. The Journal of Thoracic and Cardiovascular Surgery. 1961;**42**:722-734

[133] Wagenvoort CA, Wagenvoort N, Draulans-Noë Y. Reversibility of plexogenic pulmonary arteriopathy following banding of the pulmonary artery. The Journal of Thoracic and Cardiovascular Surgery. 1984;**87**:876-886

[134] Sakao S, Taraseviciene-Stewart L, Lee JD, Wood K, Cool CD, Voelkel NF. Initial apoptosis is followed by increased proliferation of apoptosis-resistant endothelial cells. The FASEB Journal. 2005;**19**(9):1178-1180. DOI: 10.1096/fj.04-3261fje

[135] Bull TM, Golpon H, Hebbel RP, Solovey A, Cool CD, Tuder RM, et al. Circulating endothelial cells in pulmonary hypertension. Thrombosis and Haemostasis. 2003;**90**:698-703. DOI: 10.1160/TH03-04-0251

[136] Li X, Qiu J, Pan M, Zheng D, Su Y, Wei M, et al. Correlation between congenital heart disease complicated with pulmonary artery hypertension and circulating endothelial cells as well as endothelin-1. International Journal of Clinical and Experimental Pathology. 2015;**8**:10743-10751 eCollection 2015

[137] Levy M, Bonnet D, Mauge L, Celermajer DS, Gaussem P, Smadja DM. Circulating endothelial cells in refractory pulmonary hypertension in children: Markers of treatment efficacy and clinical worsening. PLoS One. 2013;**8**(6):e65114. DOI: 10.1371/journal.pone.0065114

[138] Kawut SM, Horn EM, Berekashvili KK, Widlitz AC, Rosenzweig EB, Barst RJ. von Willebrand factor independently predicts long-term survival in patients with pulmonary arterial hypertension. Chest. 2005;**128**:2355-2362. DOI: 10.1378/chest.128.4.2355

[139] Smadja DM, Mauge L, Sanchez O, Silvestre JS, Guerin C, Godier A, et al. Distinct patterns of circulating endothelial cells in pulmonary hypertension. The European Respiratory Journal. 2010;**36**:1284-1293. DOI: 10.1183/09031936.00130809

[140] Yu W, Liu Z, An S, Zhao J, et al. The endothelial-mesenchymal transition (EndMT) and tissue regeneration. Current Stem Cell Research & Therapy. 2014;**9**:196-204

[141] Bakhshi FR, Mao M, Shajahan AN, Piegeler T, Chen Z, Chernaya O, et al. Nitrosation-dependent caveolin 1 phosphorylation, ubiquitination, and degradation and its association with idiopathic pulmonary arterial hypertension. Pulmonary Circulation. 2013;**3**(4):816-830. DOI: 10.1086/674753

[142] Li Z, Wermuth PJ, Benn BS, Lisanti MP, Jimenez SA. Caveolin-1 deficiency induces spontaneous endothelial-to-mesenchymal transition in murine pulmonary endothelial cells in vitro. The American Journal of Pathology. 2013;**182**:325-331

[143] Coll-Bonfill N, Musri MM, Ivo V, Barberà JA, Tura-Ceide O. Transdifferentiation of endothelial cells to smooth muscle cells play an important role in vascular remodelling. American Journal of Stem Cells. 2015;**4**:13-21

[144] Ranchoux B, Antigny F, Rucker-Martin C, Hautefort A, Péchoux C, Bogaard HJ, et al. Endothelial-to-mesenchymal transition in pulmonary hypertension. Circulation. 2015;**131**:1006-1018. DOI: 10.1161/CIRCULATIONAHA.114.008750

[145] Hopper RK, Moonen JR, Diebold L, Cao A, Rhodes CJ, Tojais NF, et al. In pulmonary arterial hypertension,

reduced BMPR2 promotes endothelial-to-mesenchymal transition via HMGA1 and its target slug. Circulation. 2016;**133**:1783-1794. DOI: 10.1161/CIRCULATIONAHA.115.020617

[146] Díez M, Musri MM, Ferrer E, Barberà JA, Peinado VI. Endothelial progenitor cells undergo an endothelial-to-mesenchymal transition-like process mediated by TGFbetaRI. Cardiovascular Research. 2010;**88**:502-511. DOI: 10.1093/cvr/cvq236

[147] Rabinovitch M, Gamble W, Nadas AS, Miettinen OS, Reid L. Rat pulmonary circulation after chronic hypoxia: Hemodynamic and structural features. The American Journal of Physiology. 1979;**236**:H818-H827. DOI: 10.1152/ajpheart.1979.236.6.H818

[148] Adnot S, Raffestin B, Eddahibi S, Braquet P, Chabrier PE. Loss of endothelium-dependent relaxant activity in the pulmonary circulation of rats exposed to chronic hypoxia. The Journal of Clinical Investigation. 1991;**87**:155-162. DOI: 10.1172/JCI114965

[149] Murata T, Yamawaki H, Hori M, Sato K, Ozaki H, Karaki H. Hypoxia impairs endothelium-dependent relaxation in organ cultured pulmonary artery. European Journal of Pharmacology. 2001;**421**:45-53. DOI: 10.1016/s0014-2999(01)01015-9

[150] Murata T, Sato K, Hori M, Ozaki H, Karaki H. Decreased endothelial nitric-oxide synthase (eNOS) activity resulting from abnormal interaction between eNOS and its regulatory proteins in hypoxia-induced pulmonary hypertension. Journal of Biological Chemistry. 2002;**15**(277):44085-44092. 3434. DOI: 10.1074/jbc.M205934200

[151] Gratton JP, Fontana J, O'Connor DS, Garcia-Cardena G, McCabe TJ, Sessa WC. Reconstitution of an endothelial nitric-oxide synthase (eNOS), hsp90, and caveolin-1 complex in vitro. Evidence that hsp90 facilitates calmodulin stimulated displacement of eNOS from caveolin-1. The Journal of Biological Chemistry. 2000;**275**:22268-22272. DOI: 10.1074/jbc.M001644200

[152] Fike CD, Pfister SL, Slaughter JC, Kaplowitz MR, Zhang Y, Zeng H, et al. Protein complex formation with heat shock protein 90 in chronic hypoxia-induced pulmonary hypertension in newborn piglets. The American Journal of Physiology. 2010;**299**:H1190-H1204. DOI: 10.1152/ajpheart.01207.2009

[153] Murata T, Lin MI, Stan RV, Bauer PM, Yu J, Sessa WC. Genetic evidence supporting caveolae microdomain regulation of calcium entry in endothelial cells. The Journal of Biological Chemistry. 2007;**282**:16631-16643. DOI: 10.1074/jbc.M607948200

[154] Paffett ML, Naik JS, Riddle MA, Menicucci SD, Gonzales AJ, Resta TC, et al. Altered membrane lipid domains limit pulmonary endothelial calcium entry following chronic hypoxia. American Journal of Physiology—Heart and Circulatory Physiology. 2011;**301**:H1331-H1340. DOI: 10.1152/ajpheart.00980.2010

[155] Murata T, Kinoshita K, Hori M, Kuwahara M, Tsubone H, Karaki H, et al. Statin protects endothelial nitric oxide synthase activity in hypoxia-induced pulmonary hypertension. Arteriosclerosis, Thrombosis, and Vascular Biology. 2005;**25**:2335-2342. DOI: 10.1161/01.ATV.0000186184.33537.48

[156] Penaloza D, Arias-Stella J. The heart and pulmonary circulation at high altitudes: Healthy highlanders and chronic mountain sickness. Circulation. 2007;**115**:1132-1146. DOI: 10.1161/CIRCULATIONAHA.106.624544

[157] Blanco I, Piccari L, Barberà JA. Pulmonary vasculature in COPD: The silent component. Respirology.

2016;**21**:984-994. DOI: 10.1111/resp.12772

[158] Sakao S, Voelkel NF, Tatsumi K. The vascular bed in COPD: Pulmonary hypertension and pulmonary vascular alterations. European Respiratory Review. 2014;**23**:350-355. DOI: 10.1183/09059180.00007913

[159] Peinado VI, Barbera JA, Ramirez J, Gomez FP, Roca J, Jover L, et al. Endothelial dysfunction in pulmonary arteries of patients with mild COPD. The American Journal of Physiology. 1998;**274**:L908-L913. DOI: 10.1152/ajplung.1998.274.6.L908

[160] Huber LC, Soltermann A, Fischler M, Gay S, Weder W, Russi EW, et al. Caveolin-1 expression and hemodynamics in COPD patients. Open Respiratory Medicine Journal. 2009;**3**:73-78. DOI: 10.2174/1874306400903010073

[161] Carlsen J, Hasseriis Andersen K, Boesgaard S, Iversen M, Steinbrüchel D, Bøgelund AC. Pulmonary arterial lesions in explanted lungs after transplantation correlate with severity of pulmonary hypertension in chronic obstructive pulmonary disease. The Journal of Heart and Lung Transplantation. 2013;**32**:347-354. DOI: 10.1016/j.healun.2012.11.014

Chapter 2

Pathogenesis of Abdominal Aortic Aneurysm

Michael Patel, Daniel Braga, Brad Money, Andres Pirela, Adam Zybulewski, Brandon Olivieri and Robert Beasley

Abstract

Abdominal aortic aneurysms (AAAs) are encountered by many healthcare providers such as interventional radiologists, vascular surgeons, cardiologists, and general practitioners. Much effort has been placed in the screening, diagnosis, and treatment of AAA with somewhat little understanding of its pathophysiology. AAA is a complex disease typically segmented into a process of proteolysis, inflammation, and vascular smooth muscle cell (VSMC) apoptosis with oxidative stress balancing its components. AAA and other aortic syndromes such as aortic dissection share this same process. On the other hand, AAA formation and aortic pathology may be acquired through infection like in mycotic aneurysm or may be genetic in origin such as seen with Ehlers-Danlos and Marfan syndromes.

Keywords: abdominal, aortic, aneurysm, dissection, mycotic, atherosclerosis, proteolysis, inflammation, oxidative stress, VSMC apoptosis, Marfan, Ehlers-Danlos, endovascular, vascular

1. Introduction and background of AAA

Abdominal aortic aneurysm (AAA) is a complex disease comprised of multifactorial molecular processes that carry a host of players yet to be solidified in literature. Although options continue to expand in the treatment of AAA, understanding the pathophysiology is pivotal for the development of screening tests and pharmacological treatment modalities.

In this chapter, we will go beyond the clinical context of AAA and discuss the various pathologic pathways that lead to its creation. Some of these pathways overlap with other aortic pathologies such as aortic dissection as well as mycotic aneurysm. Lastly, we will discuss common genetic disorders that are predisposed to aortic aneurysm and aortic dissection.

2. Abdominal aortic aneurysm

2.1 Normal anatomy and histology

The aorta is the main artery of the body that carries oxygenated blood from the heart to the remaining major arteries of the body. It may be segmented into the thoracic aorta and abdominal aorta based on its location to the diaphragmatic hiatus.

There are three sheaths that make up the aortic wall: tunica intima, tunica media, and tunica adventitia. The intimal layer is thin and mainly composed of endothelial cells, while the tunica media is the largest component of the aortic wall and consist of elastic fibers, smooth muscle cells, and collagenous tissue. Connective tissue makes up the most outer layer called the tunica adventitia and contains small blood vessels known as the vasa vasorum, which supply the cells of the arterial wall.

An aneurysm is defined as the localized dilatation of a vessel exceeding 1.5 times the normal diameter of the vessel, which is defined as greater than 3 cm in the abdominal aorta. As the abdominal aorta dilates, it becomes prone to rupture or tearing within the layers of its wall, otherwise known as aortic dissection (AD). In AAA and AD, patients may present with low blood pressure and a tearing sensation in the chest or back. When blood rushes into the medial layer forming a new, "false" lumen, further expansion can compress the "true" lumen causing downstream ischemia.

2.2 Role of aortic atherosclerosis

Atherosclerosis is often present in the setting of aortic pathology and although no causal pathway has been established, understanding the bridge between atherosclerosis and the inflammatory response in AAA remains essential. Early atherogenesis begins with subendothelial retention of circulating lipoproteins on proteoglycans within the extracellular matrix of the arterial wall. Aggregation and oxidation of retained lipoproteins further leads to a maladaptive immune response with circulating monocytes entering the subendothelium, differentiating into macrophages, ingesting the modified lipoproteins, and transforming into the classic "foam cell." The release of cytokines in this process, such as tumor necrosis factor-α (TNF-α) and interferon-γ (IFN-γ), leads to immune cell infiltration and inflammation [1, 2].

2.3 Pathogenesis of abdominal aortic aneurysm

Much of our understanding of AAA until this point arises from histopathological studies dating back to 1972 when the "Inflammatory" variant of AAA was described [3]. Since then, the most prevalent features of studied AAA segments have demonstrated elastin degeneration, immune cell infiltration, and apoptosis of vascular smooth muscle cells (VSMCs). Although the complete pathogenesis is unknown, information from animal models, histopathological studies and genome-wide association studies (GWAS) may be used to partition this intricate process into proteolysis, inflammation, and vascular smooth muscle cell (VSMC) apoptosis. Oxidative stress appears to be a major player as well and balances different facets of AAA development and growth.

2.3.1 Proteolysis

During aneurysmal growth, significant proteolytic degradation of elastin, collagen, laminin, fibronectin, and many other extracellular matrix (ECM) proteins occurs in the arterial wall. Upregulation of proteolytic enzymes in the aortic wall is stimulated by the presence of oxidized LDL and cytokines such as TNF-α, IL-1, and IL-3 [4]. The most famous set of proteolytic enzymes are known as the matrix metalloproteinases (MMPs), which have been implicated in cancer, wound healing, and many other processes. During normal homeostasis, regulation of MMPs in the aortic wall is carried out by tissue inhibitors of MMPs (TIMPs), but a higher MMP/TIMP ratio is typically observed in aneurysms [5, 6].

Of the multiple MMPs, MMP-9 and MMP-2 are considered crucial participants in AAA and aortic dissection (AD) development, both significantly upregulated in AAA segments with MMP-9 expression correlating with aneurysm diameter. MMP-9 is derived from macrophages and neutrophils and MMP-2 is produced by smooth muscle cells and fibroblasts; together, they both balance ECM remodeling, inflammation, and VSMC apoptosis through various signaling pathways such as the MAPK (mitogen-activated protein kinase)/ERK pathway [7]. TGF-beta signaling pathways help balance MMP-2 and MMP-9 in addition to creating protection against AAA formation by increasing type I and III collagen production and upregulating protease inhibitors [8].

2.3.2 Inflammation

Innate and adaptive arms of the immune system are involved in the development and growth of AAA. Neutrophil infiltration and release of elastase induces early degradation of the ECM in the aortic wall. Elastin breakdown products trigger either pro-inflammatory or anti-inflammatory macrophages in the adventitial layer of the aortic wall. T-cell derived interferon gamma and B cells are also involved in AAA formation. B cells provide a source of immunoglobulins, complement pathway, and cytokines, which add to the complexity of AAA formation [9–11].

2.3.3 VSMC apoptosis

Necrosis and apoptosis have traditionally been deemed different mechanisms [12]. Apoptosis is considered an organized and instructed route of cell death while necrosis is regarded as an unorganized disruption of a cell with an additional immune response. With this in mind, VSMC apoptosis occurring in the tunica media of the aortic wall in AAA formation is not a recent discovery, although the exact phenomenon is not known.

In addition to a review on cell death nomenclature, Wang et al. describe receptor-interacting protein kinase 3 (RIP3) on VSMCs as a key player in a structured form of necrosis, also known as necroptosis [12]. It is believed that RIP3 mediating inflammatory cytokine production by smooth muscle cells is mediated in the aortic wall through TNF-α signaling pathways. Additionally, protein kinase C-delta (PKC) is upregulated in aneurysmal tissues which lack VSMCs and murine models have demonstrated decreased RIP3 levels in aortic tissue that lacks PKC, further validating the role of PKC in AAA formation [13, 14].

2.4 Oxidative stress

2.4.1 Defining oxidative stress

Oxidative stress is defined as cellular injury induced by reactive oxygen species (ROS) and reactive nitrogen species (RNS), taken as a combined ROS/RNS system [15]. Pathologic oxidative stress to the vasculature occurs via a multi-faceted, highly complex mechanism that is thought to occur in part by the ROS/RNS system. The ROS/RNS system is defined as a group of molecules consisting of free radicals or molecules which predispose to free radical formation. A free radical is any species that contains one or more unpaired electrons that is capable of existing independently, which makes them highly unstable and will react readily with lipids, cellular proteins, and nucleic acids [15, 16].

2.4.2 Normal pathophysiology and regulation

The production of ROS/RNS is highly regulated and occurs naturally to some degree in all normal cells due to the incomplete reduction of molecular oxygen to water during cellular respiration and within phagosomes of phagocytic cells (chiefly neutrophils and macrophages) [15]. ROS/RNS are typically short-lived, owing to their instability and prompt removal/inactivation by endogenous cellular antioxidants and antioxidant enzymes such as catalase, glutathione peroxidase, and superoxide dismutase. Dysregulation occurs when ROS/RNS production exceeds clearance.

2.4.3 The various ROS/RNS entities and their chemical reactions

The principal ROS/RNS involved in cellular injury include superoxide, hydrogen peroxide, hydroxyl radicals, and peroxynitrite. These entities mediate vascular damage either directly or indirectly by conversion to more reactive substances [15, 16].

a. *Hydrogen peroxide.* Hydrogen peroxide (H_2O_2) is the most abundant non-radical oxidant and is formed mostly from superoxide dismutase acting on superoxide radicals [16]. In and of itself it is stable in configuration, weakly oxidizing, and can cross cellular membranes. In the presence of transitional metallic elements such as iron (Fe), hydrogen peroxide can decompose into a highly reactive and unstable hydroxyl radical (OH) in a process known as the Fenton reaction. In the Fenton reaction, peroxide is removed via conversion to H_2O and O_2 via catalase and glutathione peroxidase. Furthermore, hydrogen peroxide can be broken down into far more reactive species. For example, hydrogen peroxide will react with NO to form peroxynitrite ($ONOO^-$), a potent mediator of vascular damage. Peroxynitrite causes inactivation of enzymes by oxidation and nitration, MMP induction with subsequent vascular connective tissue breakdown, and lipid peroxidation [15–17].

b. *NADPH oxidase*. NADPH oxidase, also known as "Phagocyte Oxidase," is a well-known enzyme encoded by the NOX gene family. The NOX family is made up of multiple protein subunits that collectively oxidize nicotaminide-adenine dinucleotide phosphate (NADPH) to reduce molecular dioxygen (O_2) into the superoxide anion ($O_2^{\bullet-}$) [15, 16]. In combination with myeloperoxidase and other enzymes, NADPH oxidase is required in the oxidative destruction of microbes via phagocytosis, classically known as the "respiratory burst." In comparison to the oxidative stress in AAA, the respiratory burst occurs within the contents of a phagolysosome, so the host cell contents are protected from the ROS that are generated. Since phagocytic cells such as macrophages are also strongly implicated in the inflammatory response associated with pathology of the aortic vessel wall, it follows that membrane-bound NADPH oxidase has been suggested as one of the predominant sources of vascular ROS linked to oxidative stress in aortic pathologies such as AAA and AD [18–20].

c. The hydroxyl radical is produced by a variety of chemical reactions involving H_2O_2, H_2O, and $O_2^{\bullet-}$. The hydroxyl radical is highly reactive and will readily react with virtually any biomolecule it encounters in a short diffusion distance (about the diameter of the typical protein) [16]. It is removed via conversion to H_2O via glutathione peroxidase and has direct damaging effects on lipoproteins and DNA.

2.4.4 Reactive nitrogen species

In addition to ROS, reactive nitrogen species (RNS) also play a role in the pathophysiology of vascular dysfunction. Nitric oxide (NO) is produced via an L-arginine precursor by nitric oxide synthases with multiple cofactors. Encoded isozymes of mammalian NOS include endothelial, neuronal, and inducible subtypes (eNOS, nNOS, and iNOS, respectively). Endothelial homeostasis rests firmly upon tight regulation of endogenous NO production, but pathologic uncoupling of NOS isozymes or IFN-γ mediated NO production by macrophages can lead to excess NO and/or ROS. Peroxynitrite ($ONOO^-$), a powerful non-radical nitrosative stressor, is formed by the reaction of $O_2^{\bullet-}$ and NO and serves as the basis for other RNS derivatives such as nitrogen dioxide (NO_2) [16, 17].

Peroxynitrite is a highly reactive proatherogenic mediator and readily reacts with protein side chains and carbon dioxide to cause cellular injury [16]. A notable example is 3-nitrotyrosine, formed by the reaction of peroxynitrite with tyrosine, which has been suggested as a local marker of oxidative stress in immunostained samples of aneurysmal aortas [19]. Additionally, Kotlarczyk et al. revealed a pathway consisting of oxidative and hemodynamic stress on the aortic wall leading to increased superoxide production and NO bioavailability. This linkage corresponded to an increased rate of asymmetric thoracic aorta dilatation in patients with bicuspid aortopathy versus their tricuspid counterparts [20].

2.4.5 Role of oxidative stress in aortic pathology

The role of oxidative stress in the pathogenesis of aortic pathologies such as aortic aneurysm involves pathologic vascular remodeling along with dysfunctional balancing of connective tissue breakdown and synthesis by VSMCs [19–21]. This is thought to occur due to several mechanisms, including ROS/RNS induced VSMC apoptosis and enhanced matrix metalloproteinase (MMP) activity, which leads to progressive weakening of the aortic wall, dilatation, and eventual aneurysm formation via the breakdown of collagen, elastin, and laminin. Oxidative stress is a major modulator of MMP formation and can disrupt the corresponding balance of TIMPs that are otherwise crucial to the structural integrity of the extracellular matrix of the arterial wall [21, 22].

Additionally, ROS can disrupt VSMC proliferation via a mechanism linked to the relative local redox microenvironment concentrations of hydrogen peroxide and lipid hydroperoxides [16, 18, 23]. Hydrogen peroxide is involved in various pathways and serves as a mediator of vascular inflammation, upregulating various chemotactic and adhesion molecules such as ICAM-1, IL-8, and P-selectin which facilitate leukocyte migration into the aortic wall. In a study of patients undergoing elective infrarenal AAA repair, tissue samples of aneurysmal aortic segments demonstrated superoxide levels 2.5 times that of adjacent non-aneurysmal aortic segments, as well as increased expression and activity of NADPH oxidase [18]. In addition, changes in normal local blood flow hemodynamics in aneurysmal aortas may also induce ROS production and contribute to aortic remodeling and dissection [20, 24, 25].

Xanthine oxidoreductase (XOR) is a famous complex molybdoflavin protein known to healthcare providers as a catalyzer in the terminal steps of purine degradation, and when therapeutically inhibited, a target for treatment of hyperuricemia and gout. Although XOR may be involved in the pro-inflammatory state associated with crystal formation in gout, it may have an antioxidant role when under the optimal conditions, which necessitates further studies [26].

2.5 Aortic dissection

Similar to AAA, the physiology of aortic dissection (AD) entails a complex multifactorial process consisting of proteolysis, inflammation, and VSMC apoptosis. The differentiating factor is that hemodynamic stress results in intimal tearing of the aortic wall allowing blood to rush into the medial layer. This process creates a "true" and "false" lumen that may propagate in either direction to occlude the true lumen and/or cause a variety of issues resulting in significant morbidity and mortality.

2.6 Mycotic aneurysm

A mycotic aortic aneurysm is characterized by a local, irreversible dilatation of the aorta which is secondary to a direct bacterial or fungal inoculation of the vessel wall. The term mycotic aneurysm is actually a misnomer, as these "infective" aneurysms are most commonly bacterial in nature and fungal to a lesser extent. Staphylococcus and Salmonella species are the two most commonly cultured organisms in mycotic aneurysms, however, improved bacteriologic techniques have led to the detection of anaerobic bacteria (mostly Bacteroides, and Clostridium spp.). Mycotic aneurysms are rare as they only represent 1–2.6% of all aortic aneurysms [27, 28].

The formation of mycotic aneurysms is initiated by a microbial induced pro-inflammatory cascade of cytokines, such as TNF-α, IL-1, IL-6, invading the aortic vessel wall [28]. The recruitment of inflammatory cells within the vessel causes functional changes to VSMCs and endothelial cells with subsequent loss of integrity in the tunica media. This intense cytokine cascade causes mycotic aneurysms to progress more rapidly and aggressively than inflammatory aneurysms and thus have a higher mortality rate when compared [29].

Mycotic aneurysms most commonly affect diseased aortic endothelium in the setting of bacteremia and may present as nonspecific back pain or abdominal pain depending on the location of the lesion. Patients will typically be febrile, indicating a systemic infection, and lab values will show signs of leukocytosis and elevated ESR. Importantly, Gram negative organisms tend to cause a more virulent arterial infection than Gram positive bacteria, which makes the resultant aneurysm even more prone to rupture and further increases the risk of mortality [30–32].

Treatment of mycotic aneurysm focuses on empiric antibiotic therapy while waiting for blood culture susceptibility panel with individualized duration, surgical excision with wide debridement of infected tissues, and revascularization as needed.

2.7 Screening and diagnosis of AAA

The primary role of AAA screening and surveillance is mortality reduction, primarily through one-time and/or periodic non-invasive imaging. The initial workup of any aortic pathology begins with a focused history and physical examination. Classically, AAA may present with a pulsatile epigastric abdominal mass, but many patients are asymptomatic and lack this finding. However, the physical exam may assist in identifying more distal aneurysmal disease, particularly those occurring in the femoropopliteal distribution, which may be predictive of coexisting AAA. The physical examination is also crucial to determine a patient's baseline status in terms of perioperative risk with regards to a future surgical or endovascular intervention [33]. A number of serum biomarkers and genetic factors are known to be associated with AAA, and despite being an exciting area of developing research, the prognostic and diagnostic value of these factors has not yet been validated clinically, and therefore do not yet play a significant role in the diagnosis and management of AAA [33].

2.7.1 Screening

Ultrasound (US) and computed tomography (CT) angiography are the two primary imaging modalities used for AAA and are both highly accurate and reproducible. Transabdominal US is relatively inexpensive and can be performed in minutes without the use of ionizing radiation or iodinated contrast media. US carries a sensitivity and specificity approaching 100% in asymptomatic patients with AAA, making it the modality of choice for AAA screening and surveillance. Both the Society for Vascular Surgery (SVS) and the US Preventive Services Task Force (USPSTF) recommend a one-time screening ultrasound for AAA in men or women 65–75 years of age with a history of tobacco use [33, 34]. Various additional recommendations exist for that of first-degree relatives of those presenting with AAA, follow-up US examinations based on initial aortic diameter at initial screening, and screening in non-smokers or females, but these recommendations are supported by lower-level data or are of unclear benefit. Obesity, overlying bowel gas, and user dependence are recognized limitations ultrasound evaluation for AAA, and US may underestimate AAA size by 2 mm [33, 34]. However, limitations are invariably offset by the aforementioned benefits, and US can be useful evaluating other causes of abdominal pain, particularly in the emergent setting, resulting in a reduction in time to diagnosis and treatment. When AAA repair is indicated in an otherwise stable patient, CT offers more precise pre-operative planning via multiplanar orthogonal measurements.

2.7.2 Surveillance

Aside from baseline screening, AAA surveillance also plays a significant role in mortality reduction, by monitoring changes in AAA size over time and subsequent timely identification of patients whose risk of rupture begins to approach or outweigh the risks of intervention. Despite multiple large-scale clinical research trials comparing AAA size versus risk of rupture, vascular and radiology literature has yet to produce a single unifying surveillance parameter, but several evidence-based criteria allow patients to be safely observed over time despite a relatively small background risk of rupture. The SVS recently provided updated guidelines for the surveillance of patients with AAA, including recommended surveillance imaging at 3-year intervals for patients with AAA between 3.0 and 3.9 cm in diameter, 12-month intervals for 4.0–4.9 cm, and 6-month intervals for 5.0 and 5.4 cm [33]. The American College of Radiology (ACR) appropriateness criteria designates duplex ultrasound of the aorta/abdomen, CTA of the abdomen and pelvis with intravenous contrast, or MRA of the abdomen and pelvis with intravenous contrast as "usually appropriate" (a rating of 7, 8, or 9) for surveillance of asymptomatic AAA without previous repair [35].

The remaining aortic pathologies, including that of aortic dissection, present with a wide range of clinical, laboratory, and imaging findings, and therefore are similarly evaluated with CT or CT angiography for prompt diagnosis.

2.8 Treatment of AAA

2.8.1 Medical therapy

Hypertensive disease is the main major risk factor for aortic thoracic disease with genetic predisposition as second major risk factor [36, 37]. Although, this notion is based on studies mostly including Marfan disease patients [38]. For patients with asymptomatic AA, anti-hypertensive therapy with beta blockers is recommended for blood pressure control with the goal being to limit aortic wall expansion. Angiotensin converting enzyme inhibitors or angiotensin receptor blockers (ARBs) are preferred as well due to their role as modifiers of inflammatory mediators and by decreasing vascular smooth muscle apoptosis [38, 39].

Beta blockers have been the traditional treatment for thoracic aortic disease. It was originally demonstrated more than 70 years ago when turkeys eating sweet pea seed, *Lathyrus odoratus*, which contains the lysis oxidase inhibitor, B-aminopropionitrile, die of acute aortic dissections. The beta blocker propranolol was found to decrease deaths from dissection in B-aminopropionitrile fed turkeys [40–43]. Beta-blockers such as propranolol benefit the aortic wall through negative inotropic and chronotropic effects. Through these effects, the elastic fibers of the wall are protected from further damage and is further supported by reduction in left ventricular pressure of the heart and heart rate [44]. However, the benefit of beta-adrenergic blockade is better established in aortic dissection than in AAA because beta blockers provide theoretical benefit on blood pressure and left ventricular pressure reduction [45].

Angiotensin converting enzyme inhibition may have a beneficial role by modifying inflammatory mediators and decreasing vascular smooth muscle apoptosis. Angiotensin receptor blockers such as Losartan have been shown to prevent expansion of aneurysms by downregulation of transforming growth factor B [38, 46, 47]. Angiotensin II type 1 receptor blockade within the renin-angiotensin-aldosterone system causes a decrease in TGF-B signaling further reducing levels of intracellular mediators within the TGF-B signaling cascade, such as phosphorylated SMAD [37, 48]. By this mechanism, there is a reduced proliferation of vascular smooth-muscle cells, fibrosis, and expression of matrix metalloproteinases [49]. Overactivation of the angiotensin II type 2 receptor pathway by ARBs causes antiproliferative and anti-inflammatory effects that are beneficial in aortic wall homeostasis [50]. In contrast, ACE inhibitors limit the production of angiotensin II, producing a negative effect on Angiotensin II type 1 and type 2 receptor pathways which do not influence alternative mechanisms [46].

Medical treatment with statins (3-hydroxy-3-methylglutaryl-coenzyme A reductase inhibitors) power many of the inflammatory pathways of the formation of aortic aneurysms. Statins provide a protective effect by inhibition of matrix metalloproteinases (MMPs) and plasminogen activator due to the aforementioned proteolytic enzymes involved in the pathophysiology of aortic aneurysm formation [39, 51, 52].

2.8.2 Surgical and endovascular treatment

Historically, abdominal aortic aneurysm was treated with open surgical repair once aneurysmal growth reached a certain size or rate. Recent advancements have allowed endovascular repair to be used as the primary modality of repair with open surgical repair reserved for emergency/unconventional situations.

3. Genetic etiologies of aortic aneurysms and dissections

Genetics play an important role in the pathogenesis of various diseases. While multifactorial processes have been described in the development of AAA and AD, there are two Mendelian disorders which may lead to AAA or AD, Marfan syndrome and Ehlers-Danlos syndrome (EDS). Both have been connected to the development of AAs and ADs lacking classic risk factors such as smoking, hypertension, and old age. By definition, both of these syndromes result from mutations in a single gene and inheritance pattern. Overall, both Marfan syndrome and EDS share deleterious effects on connective tissues in the body which consequently have major ramifications on the integrity of major blood vessels.

3.1 Ehlers-Danlos syndrome

Ehlers-Danlos syndromes (EDS) are a rare group of inherited disorders of collagen which ultimately impair the integrity of the extracellular matrix of supporting structures such as connective tissues. Clinically, people with EDS usually feature remarkable hyperelastic skin, hypermobile joints, and often a bleeding diathesis. At least six clinical and genetic variants of EDS have been established and they all share a generalized defect in collagen, including abnormalities in its structure, synthesis, secretion and degradation.

In this discussion, the vascular subtype of EDS, previously referred to as type IV EDS, is the focus of this section. The vascular subtype of EDS (vEDS) is manifested from a key mutation affecting the COL3A1 gene, which subsequently causes deficient synthesis of type III procollagen. The diagnosis of vEDS is made from major and minor clinical criteria and can be confirmed by abnormalities in procollagen production as seen in protein gel electrophoresis and molecular genetic testing.

3.1.1 Epidemiology of EDS

The incidence of vEDS is roughly 1:100,000 with a total of 1500 affected individuals in the United States having been identified on the basis of biochemical and genetic testing and analysis of family pedigrees [53].

3.1.2 Molecular genetics of EDS

The COL3A1 gene is found on chromosome locus 2q32.2 and encodes for type III pro-collagen. The COL3A1 is estimated to be over 44 kb in size [54]. The vEDS subtype is inherited in an autosomal dominant pattern.

3.1.3 Pathogenesis of EDS

Type III collagen is extremely prevalent in skin, vessel walls and reticular fibers of most tissues such as the lungs, liver, and spleen. Mutations in the COL3A1 gene responsible for vEDS can take various forms. These include point mutations, deletions, insertions, splicing mutations, and missense mutations. The most common genetic mutation associated with vEDS is a missense mutation of a crucial glycine residue in the triple helical domain of the alpha-1 (III)-chains of type III procollagen. The mutation almost always occurs in a particular region of the protein that is used to bind to other collagen proteins. Three collagen proteins always bind together into a trimer, which is required for collagen functionality; when not bound in a trimer, collagen is useless, as it cannot provide functional or structural support [55].

The most common missense mutation recognized in the literature is a substitution of glycine to glutamic acid or lysine (Glu>Lys), both leading to the production of a defective polypeptide and disrupted (Gly-X-Y)n collagen motif [56]. This leads to the development of severely malformed collagen fibrils and reticulin fibers in the extracellular matrix of dermal and arterial tissues.

Type III procollagen is a major structural protein in hollow organs and vessel walls. An altered structure of the protein makes it dysfunctional in large elastic arteries such as the aorta causing them to be more prone to rupture or dissection. The mechanisms by which mutant type III collagen molecules create vascular fragility are not well understood in humans, though clinically vEDS is characterized by weakness of tissues rich in type III collagen, such as blood vessels, thus predisposing them to aneurysm and dissection [57].

3.2 Marfan syndrome

Marfan syndrome is caused by an inherited mutation of the FBN1 gene coding for the extracellular glycoprotein Fibrillin-1. The mutation in FBN1 initiates instability of connective tissue extracellular matrix, manifesting broadly as changes to the skeleton, eyes, and cardiovascular system. There have been more than 1800 distinct causative mutations in the FBN1 gene which complicates the diagnosis by DNA sequencing alone. As a result, the diagnosis of Marfan syndrome is mainly based on clinical findings. Classically you will see ectopia lentis, tall stature with coinciding arachnodactyly, and hyperlaxity of joints.

3.2.1 Epidemiology of Marfan syndrome

The prevalence of Marfan syndrome is estimated to be 1 in 5000. According to National Human Genome Research Institute, roughly 75% of cases are familial and the remaining 25% of cases are a result of a new (de novo) mutation in the FBN1 gene. In a 2015 study involving 412 people confirmed as having Marfan syndrome, the median age at diagnosis is found to be 19.0 years [58].

3.2.2 Molecular genetic of Marfan syndrome

Fibrillin-1 is encoded for by the FBN1 gene (chromosome locus 15q21) which is estimated to be 235 kb in size [59]. Marfan syndrome is inherited in an autosomal dominant pattern.

3.2.3 Pathogenesis of Marfan syndrome

Fibrillin-1 is secreted by fibroblasts, is modified post-translationally by glycosylation, and is the major component of microfibrils found in the extracellular matrix of connective tissue. Microfibrils are widely distributed in the body, more specifically they are abundant in the aorta, ligaments, and the ciliary zonules that support the ocular lens. This distribution of microfibrils gives rise to the unique clinical presentation classically known as Marfanoid habitus.

More recently, microfibril-associated glycoprotein 4 (MFAP4) has been linked to the pathogenesis of Marfan syndrome. Yin et al. using a glycoproteomic analysis of aortic extracellular matrix in Marfan patients, found an increased and more diverse N-glycosylation of MFAP4 in patients with Marfan syndrome compared with control patients. Most importantly in our discussion of AA and AD, this increased N-glycosylation was particularly in the aneurysmal stages [60, 61].

The defective Fibrillin-1 protein and subsequent faulty microfibrils are fundamental in the progression to an aortic aneurysm or an aortic dissection seen in Marfan syndrome. Not only do microfibrils provide structural integrity of specific organ systems, but they also provide a scaffold for elastogenesis in elastic tissues, most notably in elastic arteries such as the aorta [62]. In a way, malfunctioning FBN1 gene inserts malware into microfibrils, thus dismantling the scaffold needed for elastogenesis. This defective elasticity in the tunica media of elastic arteries such as the aorta weakens the vessel wall predisposing to early aneurysm. Weakening of the media also predisposes to any intimal tear, which may initiate an intramural hematoma that cleaves the layers of the media to produce aortic dissection.

Interestingly, the loss of microfibrils also gives rise to abnormal and excessive activation of transforming growth factor-B (TGF-B). Normally sequestered by well-functioning microfibrils, excessive TGF-B signaling has deleterious effects on both vascular smooth muscle development and the overall integrity of the extracellular matrix at a cellular level. Excessive TGF-B signaling in the adventitia of large elastic arteries causes increased deposition of weak fibrotic tissue leading to aneurysm development [58].

4. Conclusion

The pathogenesis of AAA formation is complex and multidimensional. The traditional atherosclerotic or inflammatory variant of AAA may be segmented into a process of proteolysis, inflammation, and VSMC apoptosis. Oxidative stress acts as a fulcrum throughout this process which is also involved in other acquired aortic pathologies such as mycotic aneurysm and aortic dissection. Classically, aortic pathology is affiliated with connective tissue disorders like seen in Marfan and Ehlers-Danlos syndromes. With further studies and eventual development, the understanding of AAA formation as well as other aortic pathologies will lead to additional treatment tools for vascular specialists and other healthcare providers alike.

Author details

Michael Patel*, Daniel Braga, Brad Money, Andres Pirela, Adam Zybulewski, Brandon Olivieri and Robert Beasley
Mount Sinai Medical Center, Nova Southeastern University College of Osteopathic Medicine, Miami, FL, USA

*Address all correspondence to: michaelpatel813@gmail.com

References

[1] Falk E. Pathogenesis of atherosclerosis. Journal of the American College of Cardiology. 2006;**47**(8):C9-C12

[2] Maguire EM, Pearce SWA, Xiao R, Oo AY, Xiao Q. Matrix metalloproteinase in abdominal aortic aneurysm and aortic dissection. Pharmaceuticals (Basel). 2019;**12**(3):2-10

[3] Walker DI, Bloor K, Williams G, Gillie I. Inflammatory aneurysms of the abdominal aorta. The British Journal of Surgery. 1972;**59**(8):609-614

[4] Abdul-hussien H, Soekhoe RG, Weber E, et al. Collagen degradation in the abdominal aneurysm: A conspiracy of matrix metalloproteinase and cysteine collagenases. The American Journal of Pathology. 2007;**170**(3):809-817

[5] Nagase H, Visse R, Murphy G. Structure and function of matrix metalloproteinases and TIMPs. Cardiovascular Research. 2006;**69**(3):562-573

[6] Freestone T, Turner RJ, Coady A, Higman DJ, Greenhalgh RM, Powell JT. Inflammation and matrix metalloproteinases in the enlarging abdominal aortic aneurysm. Arteriosclerosis, Thrombosis, and Vascular Biology. 1995;**15**(8):1145-1151

[7] Davis V, Persidskaia R, Baca-regen L, et al. Matrix metalloproteinase-2 production and its binding to the matrix are increased in abdominal aortic aneurysms. Arteriosclerosis, Thrombosis, and Vascular Biology. 1998;**18**(10):1625-1633

[8] Yoshimura K, Aoki H, Ikeda Y, et al. Regression of abdominal aortic aneurysm by inhibition of c-Jun N-terminal kinase. Nature Medicine. 2005;**11**(12):1330-1338

[9] Hasan D, Chalouhi N, Jabbour P, Hashimoto T. Macrophage imbalance (M1 vs. M2) and upregulation of mast cells in wall of ruptured human cerebral aneurysms: Preliminary results. Journal of Neuroinflammation. 2012;**9**:222

[10] Xiong W, Zhao Y, Prall A, Greiner TC, Baxter BT. Key roles of CD4+ T cells and IFN-gamma in the development of abdominal aortic aneurysms in a murine model. Journal of Immunology. 2004;**172**(4):2607-2612

[11] Furusho A, Aoki H, Ohno-urabe S, et al. Involvement of B cells, immunoglobulins, and Syk in the pathogenesis of abdominal aortic aneurysm. Journal of the American Heart Association. 2018;**7**(6):1-10

[12] Wang Q, Liu Z, Ren J, Morgan S, Assa C, Liu B. Receptor-interacting protein kinase 3 contributes to abdominal aortic aneurysms via smooth muscle cell necrosis and inflammation. Circulation Research. 2015;**116**(4):600-611

[13] He S, Wang L, Miao L, et al. Receptor interacting protein kinase-3 determines cellular necrotic response to TNF-alpha. Cell. 2009;**137**(6):1100-1111

[14] Morgan S, Yamanouchi D, Harberg C, et al. Elevated protein kinase C-δ contributes to aneurysm pathogenesis through stimulation of apoptosis and inflammatory signaling. Arteriosclerosis, Thrombosis, and Vascular Biology. 2012;**32**(10):2493-2502

[15] Kumar V, Abbas AK, Aster JC. Robbins Basic Pathology. 10th ed. New York: Elsevier; 2018

[16] Stocker R, Keaney JF Jr. Role of oxidative modifications in atherosclerosis. Physiological Reviews. 2004;**84**(4):1381-1478. DOI: 10.1152/physrev.00047.2003. Review

[17] Pacher P, Beckman JS, Liaudet L. Nitric oxide and peroxynitrite in health and disease. Physiological Reviews. 2007;**87**(1):315-424. DOI: 10.1152/physrev.00029.2006. Review

[18] McCormick ML, Gavrila D, Weintraub NL. Role of oxidative stress in the pathogenesis of abdominal aortic aneurysms. Arteriosclerosis, Thrombosis, and Vascular Biology. 2007;**27**(3):461-469. DOI: 10.1161/01.ATV.0000257552.94483.14. [Epub 11 January 2007]. Review

[19] Miller FJ Jr, Sharp WJ, Fang X, Oberley LW, Oberley TD, Weintraub NL. Oxidative stress in human abdominal aortic aneurysms: A potential mediator of aneurysmal remodeling. Arteriosclerosis, Thrombosis, and Vascular Biology. 2002;**22**(4):560-565. DOI: 10.1161/01.atv.0000013778.72404.30

[20] Kotlarczyk MP, Billard M, Green BR, Hill JC, Shiva S, Kelley EE, et al. Regional disruptions in endothelial nitric oxide pathway associated with bicuspid aortic valve. Annals of Thoracic Surgery. 2016. [Epub ahead of print]

[21] Guzik B, Sagan A, Ludew D, Mrowiecki W, Chwała M, Bujak-Gizycka B, et al. Mechanisms of oxidative stress in human aortic aneurysms-association with clinical risk factors for atherosclerosis and disease severity. International Journal of Cardiology. 2013;**168**(3):2389-2396. DOI: 10.1016/j.ijcard.2013.01.278. [Epub 15 March 2013]

[22] Rajagopalan S, Meng XP, Ramasamy S, Harrison DG, Galis ZS. Reactive oxygen species produced by macrophage-derived foam cells regulate the activity of vascular matrix metalloproteinases in vitro. Implications for atherosclerotic plaque stability. The Journal of Clinical Investigation. 1996;**98**(11):2572-2579. DOI: 10.1172/JCI119076

[23] Li WG, Miller FJ Jr, Zhang HJ, Spitz DR, Oberley LW, Weintraub NL. H(2)O(2)-induced O(2) production by a non-phagocytic NAD(P)H oxidase causes oxidant injury. The Journal of Biological Chemistry. 2001;**276**(31):29251-29256. DOI: 10.1074/jbc.M102124200. [Epub 17 May 2001]

[24] De Keulenaer GW, Chappell DC, Ishizaka N, Nerem RM, Alexander RW, Griendling KK. Oscillatory and steady laminar shear stress differentially affect human endothelial redox state: Role of a superoxide-producing NADH oxidase. Circulation Research. 1998;**82**(10):1094-1101. DOI: 10.1161/01.res.82.10.1094

[25] Nakahashi TK, Hoshina K, Tsao PS, Sho E, Sho M, Karwowski JK, et al. Flow loading induces macrophage antioxidative gene expression in experimental aneurysms. Arteriosclerosis, Thrombosis, and Vascular Biology. 2002;**22**(12):2017-2022. DOI: 10.1161/01.atv.0000042082.38014.ea

[26] Kelley EE. Dispelling dogma and misconceptions regarding the most pharmacologically targetable source of reactive species in inflammatory disease, xanthine oxidoreductase. Archives of Toxicology. 2015;**89**(8):1193-1207

[27] Brook I. Anaerobic bacteria as a cause of mycotic aneurysm of the aorta: Microbiology and antimicrobial therapy. Current Cardiology Reviews. 2009;**5**(1):36-39. DOI: 10.2174/157340309787048095

[28] Hudson JS, Hoyne DS, Hasan DM. Inflammation and human cerebral aneurysms: Current and future treatment prospects. Future Neurology. 2013;**8**(6):3-8. DOI: 10.2217/fnl.13.40

[29] Thompson MM, Boyle J. Oxford Textbook of Vascular Surgery. Oxford, United Kingdom: Oxford University Press; 2016

[30] Sekar N. Primary aortic infections and infected aneurysms. Annals of Vascular Diseases. 2010;**3**(1):24-27. DOI: 10.3400/avd.AVDctiia09001

[31] Kim YW. Infected aneurysm: Current management. Annals of Vascular Diseases. 2010;**3**(1):7-15. DOI: 10.3400/avd.AVDctiia09003

[32] Laohapensang K, Rutherford RB, Arworn S. Infected aneurysm. Annals of Vascular Diseases. 2010;**3**(1):16-23. DOI: 10.3400/avd.AVDctiia09002

[33] Chaikof EL, Dalman RL, Eskandari MK, Jackson BM, Lee WA, Mansour MA, et al. The Society for Vascular Surgery practice guidelines on the care of patients with an abdominal aortic aneurysm. Journal of Vascular Surgery. 2018;**67**(1):2-77.e2. DOI: 10.1016/j.jvs.2017.10.044

[34] Final Update Summary: Abdominal Aortic Aneurysm: Screening. U.S. Preventive Services Task Force, Rockville, MD, U.S.A; March 2017

[35] Collard M, Sutphin PD, Kalva SP, Majdalany BS, et al. American college of radiology appropriateness criteria: Abdominal aortic aneurysm follow-up (without repair). American College of Radiology. May 2019;**16**(5S):S2-S6. [Accessed: 30 September 2019]

[36] Brownstein A, Ziganshin B, Kuivaniemi H, Body S, Bale A, Elefteriades J. Genes associated with thoracic aortic aneurysm and dissection. Aorta. 2017;**05**(01):11-20. DOI: 10.12945/j.aorta.2017.17.003

[37] Chan KK, Rabkin SW. Increasing prevalence of hypertension among patients with thoracic aorta dissection: Trends over eight decades—A structured meta-analysis. American Journal of Hypertension. 2014;**27**(7):907-917. DOI: 10.1093/ajh/hpt293

[38] Yetman AT, Bornemeier RA, McCrindle BW. Usefulness of enalapril versus propranolol or atenolol for prevention of aortic dilation in patients with the Marfan syndrome. The American Journal of Cardiology. 2005;**95**(9):1125-1127. DOI: 10.1016/j.amjcard.2005.01.032

[39] Elefteriades JA. Does medical therapy for thoracic aortic aneurysms really work? Are β-blockers truly indicated? PRO. Cardiology Clinics. 2010;**28**(2):255-260. DOI: 10.1016/j.ccl.2010.02.016

[40] Bachhuber TE, Lalich JJ, Angevine DM, Schilling ED, Strong FM. Lathyrus factor activity of beta-aminopropionitrile and related compounds. Proceedings of the Society for Experimental Biology and Medicine. 1955;**89**(2):294-297

[41] Milewicz DM, Ramirez F. Therapies for thoracic aortic aneurysms and acute aortic dissections. Arteriosclerosis, Thrombosis, and Vascular Biology. 2019;**39**(2):126-136. DOI: 10.1161/ATVBAHA.118.310956

[42] Simpson CF, Kling JM, Palmer RF. The use of propranolol for the protection of turkeys from the development of β-aminopropionitrile-induced aortic ruptures. Angiology. 1968;**19**(7):414-418

[43] Simpson CF. Sotalol for the protection of turkeys from the development of β-aminopropionitrile-induced aortic ruptures. British Journal of Pharmacology. 1972;**45**(3):385-390

[44] Shores J, Berger KR, Murphy EA, Pyeritz RE. Progression of aortic dilatation and the benefit of long-term β-adrenergic blockade in Marfan's

syndrome. The New England Journal of Medicine. 1994;**330**(19):1335-1341

[45] Gersony DR, McClaughlin MA, Jin Z, Gersony WM. The effect of beta-blocker therapy on clinical outcome in patients with Marfan's syndrome: A meta-analysis. International Journal of Cardiology. 2007;**114**(3):303-308. DOI: 10.1016/j.ijcard.2005.11.116

[46] Brooke BS, Habashi JP, Judge DP, Patel N, Loeys B, Dietz HC. Angiotensin II blockade and aortic-root dilation in Marfan's syndrome. The New England Journal of Medicine. 2008;**358**(26):2787-2795. DOI: 10.1056/NEJMoa0706585

[47] Bowman MAH, Eagle KA, Milewicz DM. Update on clinical trials of losartan with and without β-blockers to block aneurysm growth in patients with Marfan syndrome: A review. JAMA Cardiology. 2019;**4**(7):702-707

[48] Lim DS, Lutucuta S, Bachireddy P, et al. Angiotensin II blockade reverses myocardial fibrosis in a transgenic mouse model of human hypertrophic cardiomyopathy. Circulation. 2001;**103**(6):789-791

[49] Neptune ER, Frischmeyer PA, Arking DE, et al. Dysregulation of TGF-β activation contributes to pathogenesis in Marfan syndrome. Nature Genetics. 2003;**33**(3):407-411

[50] Wu L, Iwai M, Nakagami H, et al. Effect of angiotensin II type 1 receptor blockade on cardiac remodeling in angiotensin II type 2 receptor null mice. Arteriosclerosis, Thrombosis, and Vascular Biology. 2002;**22**(1):49-54

[51] Stein LH, Berger J, Tranquilli M, Elefteraides JA. Effect of statin drugs on thoracic aortic aneurysms. The American Journal of Cardiology. 2013;**112**(8):1240-1245

[52] Schmoker JD, McPartland KJ, Fellinger EK, et al. Matrix metalloproteinase and tissue inhibitor expression in atherosclerotic and nonatherosclerotic thoracic aortic aneurysms. The Journal of Thoracic and Cardiovascular Surgery. 2007;**133**(1):155-161

[53] Rodwell VW, Bender DA, Botham KM, Kennelly PJ, Weil PA. Harpers Illustrated Biochemistry. 31st ed. New York: McGraw-Hill Education; 2018

[54] Adam MP, Ardinger HH, Pagon RA, et al., editors. GeneReviews® [Internet]. Seattle, WA: University of Washington, Seattle; 1993-2019

[55] Mizuno K, Boudko S, Engel J, Bächinger HP. Vascular Ehlers-Danlos syndrome mutations in type III collagen differently stall the triple helical folding. The Journal of Biological Chemistry. 2013;**288**(26):19166-19176. DOI: 10.1074/jbc.M113.462002. [Epub 03 May 2013]

[56] Ghali N, Baker D, Brady AF, Burrows N, Cervi E, Cilliers D, et al. Atypical COL3A1 variants (glutamic acid to lysine) cause vascular Ehlers-Danlos syndrome with a consistent phenotype of tissue fragility and skin hyperextensibility. Genetics in Medicine. 2019;**21**(9):2081-2091. DOI: 10.1038/s41436-019-0470-9. [Epub 06 March 2019]

[57] D'hondt S, Guillemyn B, Syx D, Symoens S, De Rycke R, Vanhoutte L, et al. Type III collagen affects dermal and vascular collagen fibrillogenesis and tissue integrity in a mutant Col3a1 transgenic mouse model. Matrix Biology. 2018;**70**:72-83. DOI: 10.1016/j.matbio.2018.03.008. [Epub March 2018]

[58] Groth KA, Hove H, Kyhl K, Folkestad L, Gaustadnes M, Vejlstrup N, et al. Prevalence, incidence, and age at diagnosis in Marfan Syndrome. Orphanet Journal of Rare Diseases.

2015;**10**:153. DOI: 10.1186/s13023-015-0369-8

[59] Liu W, Schrijver I, Brenn T, Furthmayr H, Francke U. Multi-exon deletions of the FBN1 gene in Marfan syndrome. BMC Medical Genetics. 2001;**2**:11. [Epub 24 October 2001]

[60] Yin 殷晓科 X, Wanga S, Fellows AL, Barallobre-Barreiro J, Lu R, Davaapil H, et al. Glycoproteomic analysis of the aortic extracellular matrix in Marfan patients. Arteriosclerosis, Thrombosis, and Vascular Biology. 2019;**39**(9):1859-1873. DOI: 10.1161/ATVBAHA.118.312175. [Epub 18 July 2019]

[61] Mecham RP, Gibson MA. The Microfibril-Associated Glycoproteins (MAGPs) and the Microfibrillar Niche. Matrix Biology. 2015;**47**:13-33. DOI: 10.1016/j.matbio.2015.05.003

[62] Halper J, Kjaer M. Basic components of connective tissues and extracellular matrix: Elastin, fibrillin, fibulins, fibrinogen, fibronectin, laminin, tenascins and thrombospondins. Advances in Experimental Medicine and Biology. 2014;**802**:31-47. DOI: 10.1007/978-94-007-7893-1_3. Review

Chapter 3

The Importance of Autophagy and Proteostasis in Metabolic Cardiomyopathy

María Cristina Islas-Carbajal, Ana Rosa Rincón-Sánchez, Cesar Arturo Nava-Valdivia and Claudia Lisette Charles-Niño

Abstract

Metabolic cardiomyopathy and other heart disorders are associated with proteostasis derailment and subsequent autophagy. Proteostasis is a process of protein homeostasis, and autophagy is a mechanism of self-degradation for surviving cells facing stressful conditions. Metabolic challenges have been linked to excess reactive oxygen species. Cardiomyocyte proteotoxicity, an important underlying pathologic mechanism in cardiac disease, is characterized by chronic accumulation of misfolded or unfolded proteins that can lead to proteotoxic formation or aggregation of soluble peptides. Autophagic processes are mediated by the ubiquitin-proteasome and autophagy-lysosome systems, fundamental for cardiac adaptation to physiological and pathological stress. Cellular proteostasis alterations in cardiomyopathy are represented by myocardial remodeling and interstitial fibrosis with reduced diastolic function and arrhythmias. Autophagy regulation may be a potential therapeutic strategy for metabolic cardiomyopathy necessary for the treatment of fibrosis and cardiac tissue remodeling alterations. Furthermore, autophagy has been shown to be active in the perimeter of cardiovascular fibrotic tissue as mechanism of fibrosis recovery and scarring secondary to cell apoptosis. In the present work, we review the current knowledge on the role of autophagy and proteostasis in the pathogenesis of heart failure to resolve the ever-expanding epidemic of metabolic cardiomyopathy and heart failure associated with substantial morbidity and mortality.

Keywords: autophagy, proteostasis, cardiac hypertrophy, metabolic cardiomyopathy, myocardial interstitial fibrosis, heart failure

1. Introduction

Metabolic cardiomyopathies can be caused by disturbances in metabolism and may develop in the context of a broad spectrum of pathological conditions. These disorders include a number of inherited metabolic diseases in early childhood affecting the heart and other organs. Cardiomyopathies are associated with systemic metabolic diseases acquired during adulthood, such as metabolic syndrome, dyslipidemia, obesity, hypertension, diabetes mellitus and cardiomyopathy by alcoholism [1], which are also considered important causes of cardiovascular diseases. Furthermore, abnormal mitochondrial function related to mitochondrial ATP-producing capacity and high cardiac energy demand is linked to several of these cardiovascular diseases. The heart is a high-energy-demanding organ and mitochondria are important organelles that provide its source of cellular energy by oxidative phosphorylation; however, enzyme deficiency related to mitochondrial beta-oxidation leads to cardiac disorders. Another key point is that autophagic activity has been found to decrease with age resulting in intracellular protein aggregate accumulation, unfolded protein response activation and subsequent cardiomyocyte apoptosis, likely contributing to the accumulation of damaged macromolecules and organelles during aging. Equally important, several forms of heart failure are progressive disorders associated with substantial morbidity and mortality, and of these, cardiovascular pathologies are the leading cause of death in the elderly. Autophagy, a lysosome-mediated degradation pathway, plays a critical role in proteostasis by removing potentially toxic cytosolic protein aggregates and damaged organelles within cells [2]. Cardiomyocyte proteostasis is the gradual derailment of cellular protein homeostasis important to protein quality control [3]. The dysfunction in proteostasis leading to the accumulation of protein aggregates is the hallmark of cardiovascular disease and many chronic and age-related diseases [4].

The metabolic syndrome has become one of the most important topics in recent decades because of the marked increase in cardiovascular risk associated with the clustering of risk factors [5]. Obesity is a major independent risk factor for cardiovascular disease, including cardiac hypertrophy and heart failure. Leptin, an adipocyte-derived hormone, acts through its receptors (LepRs) on hypothalamic neurons that regulate body weight and energy homeostasis. LepRs are also expressed on cardiovascular cells, and leptin has also been shown to promote cardiomyocyte hypertrophy, endothelial proliferation, migration and angiogenesis, and fibrosis.

The effects of the mechanistic target of rapamycin (mTOR) are mediated through its activity as a central inhibitor of autophagy, a highly conserved cell survival mechanism. Cardiac hypertrophy is associated with increased energy demands, and cellular stressors like ischemia or nutrient deprivation, which result in the rapid regulation of myocardial autophagy. In this context, endothelial cells are particularly sensitive to metabolic stress, and defective or maladaptive endothelial autophagy may contribute to the rarefaction of the cardiac microvasculature during hypertrophy, a critical event in the transition toward heart failure [6]. In the present work, we review the current understanding of the role of autophagy and proteostasis in the pathogenesis of heart disease, considering the essential involvement of both degradation processes to find a novel therapeutic target to resolve the ever-expanding epidemic of metabolic cardiomyopathy and heart failure associated with significant morbidity and mortality.

2. Proteostasis

A complex proteostasis network functions to ensure the maintenance of proteostasis, consisting of molecular chaperones and proteolytic machineries and their regulators in healthy cells. Each type of these molecules with a precise amino acid sequence has important physical properties to determine specific protein structure and a three-dimensional conformation to proteins, which is important in order to regulate cellular performance and balance. Protein structures are made by the formation of peptide bonds that build the polypeptide long chains of alpha-amino acids, a common property of all proteins. Disturbed proteostasis in postmitotic cell types, such as cardiomyocytes and neurons, produces an accumulation of misfolded and aggregated proteins resulting in disease. These factors coordinate protein synthesis with polypeptide folding for the conservation of protein conformation and protein degradation. In particular, maintaining proteome balance is a challenging task against external and endogenous stresses that accumulate during chronic cardiovascular disease and aging, which lead to the decline of the proteostasis network capacity and proteome integrity [4].

2.1 Balance and integrity of the proteome

The protein flux of the cell must remain in balance to ensure proper cell and tissue function. The protein homeostasis, also known as proteostasis, leads to the accumulation of protein aggregates and it is the cause of several diseases. In view of this, protein aggregation is a common characteristic of many chronic diseases. Proteome balance is a task in defiance of external and endogenous stresses that accumulate in a lifetime, such as chronic cardiovascular diseases and aging. Moreover, regulated proteolysis mediated by proteases of damaged proteins is fundamental for protein quality control of eukaryotic cells that require the ubiquitin-proteasome system (UPS). The UPS activity can be executed by ubiquitin-protein ligases or chaperones and the first crucial step is recognition of a specific degradation signal (degron). Degrons are portions of a protein that when exposed create a signal that is recognized by target proteins to the UPS pathway [7].

From this perspective, after several steps of substrate polyubiquitylation followed by substrate unfolding and degradation, proteins with specific degrons are recognized by the proteasome and targeted for degradation.

The cellular proteome is exceedingly complex and large-scale proteomic studies have identified thousands of modification sites (common modifications include phosphorylation, ubiquitylation, methylation and acetylation) in roughly 50% of proteins in humans, the combinatorial nature of which is mostly unknown [8]. Individual proteins often exist in several modified forms and they also engage in numerous dynamically regulated protein complexes during their life cycle. It is estimated that about 100,000 distinct protein isoforms can be generated through alternative splicing from all the pool of protein-coding genes. Nonetheless, the mechanisms that underlie the dynamics, interactions, stoichiometry and turnover of most individual protein species are poorly understood at the global level [8].

2.2 Proteostasis and its network

In the cell, the proteome is a wide surveillance and regulatory network of the biogenesis process and protein degradation, which intervenes when these processes develop in a suboptimal way [8]. Proteome imbalance often results in complex and chronic diseases; therefore, it is a continuous process in order to meet the dynamic of proteomic needs of the cell [8]. In healthy cells, a complex proteostasis network (PN), comprised of molecular chaperones and proteolytic machineries and their regulators, operates to ensure the maintenance of proteostasis. These factors coordinate protein synthesis with polypeptide folding, the conservation of protein conformation and protein degradation [4]. The PN is performed by mechanisms controlling protein biosynthesis, cotranslational folding process, trafficking, neofunctionalization and degradation of proteins in vivo, among others, to maintain proteome balance and conform to the PN [9].

The proteome must have the ability to generate adequate synthesis, folding and protein expression and at the same time to detect abnormalities during this process by identifying the characteristics that force protective degradation when a component lacks quality. Human cells have more than 10^3 proteins per cell, and 5% of these are involved only in protein synthesis and turnover, and 60–80% of the etiologies of some diseases are associated with misfolding proteins. Therefore, it is clear that the constantly dynamic and complex eukaryote proteome requires a tightly regulated process [10].

The description of cellular proteomes requires an understanding not only of how proteins and their multimeric assemblies are built and their mechanisms established but also of the rules that determine how proteins are selected for degradation when they are unable to assemble properly with components of cognate networks. The network is constantly regulating the proteome, but it responds to conditions of proteotoxic stress by addressing the triage decision of fold, hold or degrade [11]. Consequently, the PN is constantly regulating the proteome and influences several cellular functions by affecting their physiology and readapting through transcriptional and translational changes within the biology of the cell [10, 11].

Numerous biological pathways affecting protein synthesis, folding, misfolding, trafficking, disaggregation and degradation may adapt the PN by using proteostasis regulators that can partially correct protein impairment, resulting in human diseases by cell stress and aging. The main PN components include several modules like protein synthesis machinery and the major mammalian protein degradation: UPS that is central to the unfolding protein response (UPR), which is activated when unfolded or misassembled proteins accumulate in the endoplasmic reticulum (ER), and the armada of intra- and extracellular chaperones including proteases, which detoxify cells from nonrepairable proteins [10, 11].

The structure of a determined protein is crucial for its function; hence, molecular chaperones are important components of the PN. Chaperones and other proteins like oxidoreductases and glycosylating enzymes bind nascent proteins and assist in proper folding into the correct structure and cellular location throughout their life cycle [12].

Diverse agents modify the structure of proteins like aging, oxidative, and thermal stress or misfolding-prone mutations. In this context, misfolded, damaged, unnecessary or aggregated proteins should be degraded, or their interactions could cause cell instability. There are two major intracellular proteolysis pathways: the autophagy-lysosomal pathway and UPS [13]. The difference between these two processes is the nature of the targeted protein degradation: in the case of autophagy, it mainly acts in the cytoplasm, and for UPS, considered the main route of protein degradation in mammalian cells, it acts on both cytoplasm and nucleus [14].

A deficient PN allows the disruption of cellular membranes by damaged proteins or toxic aggregates, which interfere with cell function, and as a result, many metabolic, oncological, cardiovascular and neurodegenerative disorders could appear in the individual [15].

The UPS is a complex machine formed by numerous subunits that degrade ubiquitin-attached proteins. This proteolysis pathway is critical for the quality control of proteins by eliminating damaged proteins and also maintaining the concentration of many regulatory proteins of apoptosis, inflammation, signal transduction and cell cycle [12]. The other proteolysis pathway, autophagy that is in charge of degraded proteins, is not detected by the UPS, and it has an important role in the immune response and starvation stage [16]. Autophagy eliminates several dysfunctional cell components or catabolizes them when the cell is under starvation and stress to maintain optimal levels of energy and nutrients [12]. ROS, DNA damage or starvation activates this autoproteolysis pathway engulfing organelles in the autophagosome that are later fused with lysosomes, and by doing so, the amino acids and fatty acids produced by the catabolism of the organelles are recycled in the cytoplasm. However, three ways of delivering target proteins to the lysosome have been identified, and based on this, autophagy is classified into three distinct types: microautophagy, chaperone-mediated autophagy (CMA) and macroautophagy [16].

In microautophagy, the cellular contents are invaginated directly by the lysosome. The major cytosolic chaperone systems are HSP70 and HSP90, which are connected to the UPS pathway. The proteasome complex contains the proteolytic active sites in the core particle (20S) and the regulatory activity of the holo-complex in the regulatory particle (19S). The UPS pathway only recognizes polyubiquitination proteins, a process that requires three enzymes: E1 ubiquitin activator, E2 conjugase and E3 ligase, which act sequentially. The polyubiquitylated proteins are recognized by the core particle for their degradation by the regulatory particle (19S) [17]. Meanwhile, CMA uses the molecular chaperone, known as heat shock cognate 71 kDa protein (Hsc70), for recognition of the KFERQ sequence motif in cytosolic proteins that must be degraded, and drives them to the lysosome membrane [18]. The transmembrane receptor or docking protein is a lysosomal-associated membrane protein-2A (LAMP-2A) that transports the unfolded cytosolic proteins into the lysosome [18].

Macroautophagy involves the formation of the autophagosomes, defined as special structures that invaginate cellular contents or target proteins and then transport them to the lysosome. Besides eliminating pathogens, autophagy is also required for antigen presentation by the major histocompatibility complex (MHC) class II. The major autophagy pathway used by cells is the MHC class II [16].

2.3 Cardiomyopathy, cellular proteostasis alterations and myocardial remodeling with interstitial fibrosis

Diabetic cardiomyopathy (DC) is a specific heart muscle disease that increases the risk of heart failure and mortality in diabetic patients independent of vascular pathology. Basal level autophagy plays a housekeeping role to maintain cellular homeostasis. However, autophagy mechanisms are impaired in diabetic hearts. In this sense, diminished autophagy limits cardiac injury in type 1 diabetes and inhibited autophagy contributes to cardiac injury in type 2 diabetes. In this context, protein homeostasis is a necessity for the correct function of the cell, in other words, an interaction between protein synthesis, transport, post-translational modification and degradation [17]. However, an accumulation of defective proteins results in proteotoxicity or disturbed proteostasis. Progression of cardiovascular diseases due to proteostasis alterations has been related with interstitial fibrosis and altered myocardial remodeling. Recent evidence indicates that the progression of ventricular dysfunction may be associated with changes in the process of autophagy and impaired proteostasis.

Autophagy in the mitochondria is a necessary process for maintaining a healthy mitochondrial network, also known as mitophagy. Under pathological conditions, mitochondrial dysfunction and enhanced ROS generation associated to cardiac hypertrophy and impaired left ventricular function with increased aggregation of abnormal proteins and enlarged or collapsed mitochondria can be found, such as structural and functional remodeling with changes in composition of the extracellular matrix, which are characterized by fibrotic tissue, impaired vascular and coronary microvascular function or effects on subcellular cardiomyocyte composition (**Figure 1**). Thus, mitophagy has been shown to be essential for myocardial protection [19]. In addition, calorie restriction is sufficient to accelerate cardiac

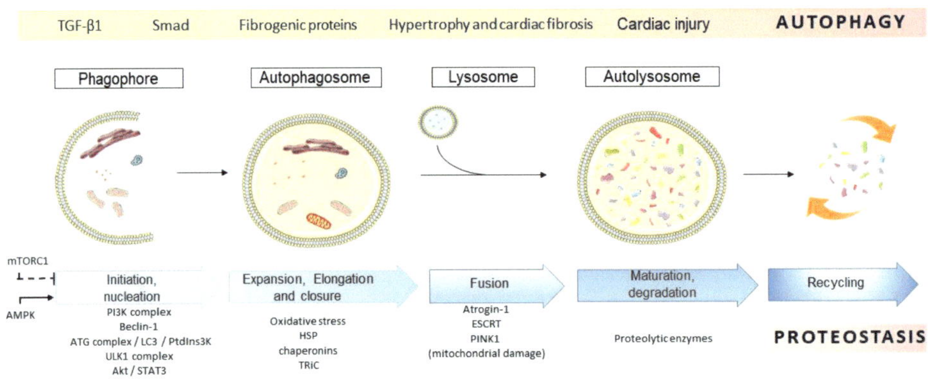

Figure 1.
Factors involved in autophagy and proteostasis in metabolic cardiomyopathy. Many proteins participate in the activation and formation of the autophagosome. TGF-β1 induces the activation of signaling pathways such as Smad, which in turn activates the formation of fibrogenic proteins such as type 1 collagen and fibronectin, and these induce hypertrophy and cardiac fibrosis generating cardiac damage and activating autophagy in cardiomyocytes. Modified of Kobayashi et al. [19].

autophagic flux and reduce mitochondrial oxidative damage in the heart, results that suggest the important role of autophagy for maintaining optimal mitochondrial structure and function [20].

Proteostasis and autophagy are related to various heart diseases; however, both mechanisms can be beneficial or harmful depending on age and pathology. From this standpoint, heart diseases linked to autophagy due to degradation of contractile heart proteins are associated with cardiac aging, inherited cardiomyopathy, diabetic cardiomyopathy (DC), atherosclerosis, heart failure (HF) and atrial fibrillation (AF) [20]. The quality of cardiomyocytes depends on the efficient elimination of damaged proteins by autophagy. The mechanism performed by chaperone proteins, particularly heat shock proteins (HSP70/HSP40/HSP110) and chaperonins like the T-complex protein 1 ring complex (TRiC), takes place to a greater extent in the heart in response to oxidative stress [21]. HSPs are found in specific protein regions to prevent aggregation; these HSPs regulate oxidative stress (OS) and metabolism and maintain proper cell proliferation. The imbalance in the degradation of damaged intracellular proteins induces aging of the heart muscle fibers as a result of OS, the deterioration of the Ca^{+2} transits and the excessive generation of ROS. This process affects remodeling, favoring hypertrophy and cardiac fibrosis [22].

In cardiomyopathies, the accumulation of incorrectly folded proteins or acquired dysfunction of protein quality control has been implicated in impaired proteostasis. The cellular function in the myocardium follows the regulation of proteostasis and autophagy in order to control the quality of new synthesized proteins and removal of unfolded/misfolded proteins. When UPS targets are too large to be degraded by the proteasome, the autophagy system must control degradation through the selection between UPS and autophagy. Among autophagy regulators, the endosomal sorting complex required for transport protein complexes (ESCRT) affects the lysosome-autophagosome fusion. Part of ESCRT is the charged multivesicular body protein 2B (CHMP2B), which is required for autophagy. The work of Zaglia et al., in 2014, identified a novel link between UPS and autophagy and showed that the muscle-specific ubiquitin ligase atrogin-1 controls turnover of the ESCRT-III family protein CHMP2B, which controls the autophagy signaling pathways [23].

Transforming growth factor β1 (TGF-β1) is an important regulator of fibrogenesis. Its expression is regulated by biochemical stimuli, as a humoral response to infections, glucose and pH [24]. Binding of TGF-β1 to specific cellular receptors, such as TGF-β type II and RII, activates phosphorylation for intracellular signaling pathways, such as Smad2 and Smad3 [25], which induce the expression of fibrogenic proteins like type I collagen and fibronectin [26]. These pathways trigger an inappropriate deposition of collagen in cardiac fibers, causing impaired heart function [27]. However, in other cell lineages, TGF-β1 is also capable of inducing autophagy, so the regulatory mechanisms between the two events are unknown [26].

Many target molecules are involved in fibrosis including the multiprotein complex formed by phosphoinositide 3-kinase class III (PI3K) dependent on Beclin 1, which regulates vesicular autophagy by activation of signaling pathways, such as Akt, and, in turn, increases the expression of TGF-β for the development of fibrosis [28]. HSP25 and alpha B-crystallin are expressed to a lesser extent in the heart; however, they fulfill the function of chaperone proteins that favor stability between actin and desmin, thus avoiding cardiotoxicity [29]. PINK1 (PTEN-induced putative kinase 1) is another protein involved in autophagy. It is located in the outer membrane of defective mitochondria, and it favors autophagy through the recruitment of the Parkin protein to depolarized mitochondria of cardiomyocytes [30].

These mechanisms can induce deregulation of autophagy by apoptosis in type II cells in cardiac tissue, which leads to the development of myocardial infarction (MI) [31]. Moreover, autophagy has been shown to be active in the perimeter of cardiovascular fibrotic tissue as a mechanism for fibrosis recovery and scarring secondary to cell apoptosis [32]. Many molecules protect against type 1 diabetes–induced cardiac dysfunction by activating autophagy. Lastly, the inhibition of autophagy has a beneficial effect on type 2 diabetes–induced cardiomyopathy [33].

2.4 Mitophagy and redox dysregulation

Cardiomyopathies as a result of excessive ROS production and protein modifications in the mitochondria involve abnormal mitochondrial function resulting in cardiac disorders due to the high energy demand of the heart through this organelle, considered as a source of cellular energy production and mitochondrial ATP production achieved by oxidative phosphorylation and beta-oxidation. As a result of mitochondrial damage, the process of autophagy, known as mitophagy, is essential for myocardial function and protection [19].

The physiological performance of endothelial nitric oxide synthase enzyme (eNOS) is important for NO production, which is dependent on L-arginine through its reaction with O_2 and the constitutive eNOS dependent on Ca^{2+}/calmodulin, as well as the cofactors (6R-)5,6,7,8-tetrahydrobiopterin (BH_4), nicotinamide adenine dinucleotide phosphate (NADPH), flavin adenine dinucleotide (FAD) and flavin mononucleotide (FMN). Nitric oxide (NO) produced by the endothelium from eNOS, which is oxidized to L-citrulline and NO, works through the transference of electrons from NADPH via FAD and FMN. Both eNOS constitutive activation events are dependent, and in caveolae, they are Ca^{2+}/calmodulin concentration dependent [34].

Under pathological situations and in the presence of uncoupled eNOS, increased OS is produced, instead of producing NO after eNOS activation due to the reaction with reduced BH_4 levels and upregulated NADPH. As a result of these cardiovascular (CV) risk factors, NO is not produced, but there is ROS production. These abnormal reactions due to CV risk factors reduce bioactive NO [34].

The biological abnormalities produced by excessive ROS production such as superoxide anion (—O_2), hydrogen peroxide (H_2O_2) and hydroxyl radical (—OH) species [35], including the rapid interaction of O_2^- with NO, result in the loss of NO bioavailability and increased production of peroxynitrite ($ONOO^-$) [34].

The harmful overproduction of these ROS and protein mitochondrial modifications as a result of impaired redox and pathological signaling in the CV system mediate regulation of the most important ion channels, transporters and kinases related to heart diseases.

These mechanisms lead to selective cardiac dysfunction and decreased energy production due to reductions in mitochondrial respiration, increased OS and defective contractile Ca^{2+} regulatory proteins. These types of changes and alterations in mitochondrial biogenesis, content and function related to an heterogeneous group of cardiovascular disease risk factors like metabolic syndrome, have been documented. Damaged mitochondria are degraded through mitophagy, the main protective function of autophagy that is for myocardial protection and the target of successful drug development emerging in the cardiovascular space. These strategies may be applied upon several redox targets, such as the membrane caveolae region where key cardiovascular redox proteins, such as eNOS, calmodulin and NADPH oxidase, among other important cardiovascular-related receptors, are located. Thus, calorie restriction is sufficient to accelerate cardiac autophagic flux to help improve mitochondrial oxidative damage and to maintain a healthy mitochondrial network [11, 18, 19].

3. Autophagy

Dr. Christian de Duve was the first to use the term "autophagy," meaning "self-eating" in Greek, at the Ciba Foundation Symposium on Lysosomes, which took place in London on February 12–14, 1963 [36]. When there is a functional decline in the cardiovascular system and aging, cardiomyocytes need a cellular control mechanism to minimize damage and prevent cardiac malfunction. In this context, autophagy may degrade and recycle long-lived proteins, cytoplasmic components and organelles [37]. The notion of autophagy as cell death is a phenomenon that has been controversial and remains mechanistically undefined. It should be noted that when autophagy promotes cell death, there is an association of autophagy with the different cell death pathways [38].

The biogenesis of an autophagosome is orchestrated by the so-called autophagy-related (ATG) proteins, which act in a hierarchical order to first generate the phagophore and then expand it into an autophagosome. The mammalian homologs of ATG1 are the uncoordinated-51-like kinases 1 and 2 (ULKA1 and ULK2) ULK complex, the ATG9A cycling system and the autophagy-specific class III phosphatidylinositol 3-kinase (PtdIns3K) complex, which are key in generating the phagophore upon induction of autophagy [39]. Besides, knockdown of EP300 and the inhibition of histone acetylases potentially induce autophagy indicating that protein deacetylation may play a role in the autophagic cascade. EP300 acetylates several autophagy-related proteins, including autophagy-related 5 (ATG5), ATG7, ATG12 and microtubule-associated protein 1 light chain 3 β (LC3). Lastly, protein deacetylation influenced by several proteins controls autophagy at diverse levels from the modification of autophagy core proteins to transcriptional factors controlling autophagic genes [39].

3.1 Autophagy basics

Autophagy is also considered an evolutionarily conserved process critical for cellular homeostasis [3]. Implication of either the pathogenesis or the response to a wide variety of diseases by autophagy has been related to the pathogenesis of various disease states and to the basic molecular pathways that regulate autophagy [40].

Basal levels of autophagy maintain cellular homeostasis, and under stress conditions, high levels of autophagy are induced. However, the pro-death role of autophagy is complicated due to the extensive cross-talk between different signaling pathways [38]. Autophagy is a process by which cytoplasmic components are sequestered in double membrane vesicles and degraded upon fusion with lysosomal compartments. Depending on the stimulus, autophagy can degrade cytoplasmic contents nonspecifically or it can target the degradation of specific cellular components. Higher eukaryotes have adopted both of these mechanisms and account for the expanding role of autophagy in various cellular processes, as well as they contribute to the variation in cellular outcomes after induction of autophagy. As the basic molecular pathways that regulate autophagy are elucidated, the relationship of autophagy to the pathogenesis of various disease states becomes apparent [40].

Autophagy is a highly conserved eukaryotic pathway responsible for the lysosomal degradation (and subsequent recycling) that is rapidly growing and elucidating an intriguing mechanistic complexity as well as a tremendous range of cargo substrates. Imbalances in proteostasis are connected to aging and multiple (age-associated) disorders [41]. Several pathologies including cardiovascular disease and stress-related disorders are associated with autophagy dysregulation. Moreover, excessive or insufficient levels of autophagic flux have been characterized in cardiomyocytes, cardiac fibroblasts, endothelial cells and vascular smooth muscle cells within the cardiovascular system [42]. Damaged and potentially cytotoxic mitochondria elicit an autophagic response termed mitophagy. Depending on the initiating stimulus, the substrate selection could differ. Thus, mitophagy takes part in physiological processes like the removal of paternal mitochondria during egg fertilization, and it is also a key process for the removal of damaged mitochondria in toxic conditions [43]. Furthermore, autophagy stimulation may result in reduced accumulation of misfolded and aggregated proteins; however, the overactivation of autophagy can trigger autophagy-mediated apoptosis.

3.2 Autophagy and heart diseases

The cardiovascular system has the ability to adapt to a wide range of environmental stresses. The myocardium itself manifests robust plasticity for both physiological and pathological stimuli. From this perspective, autophagy is an intracellular process required to maintain cardiovascular homeostasis, and it is also an evolutionarily ancient process of intracellular catabolism in response to a wide variety of stresses. In the case of postmitotic cells, where cell replacement is not an option, finely tuned quality control of cytoplasmic constituents and organelles is especially critical [41]. Mitochondrial DNA has an important role at inducing and maintaining inflammation in the heart that escapes from autophagy. These autophagic mechanisms degrade damaged mitochondria through fusion of autophagosomes and lysosomes. Lastly, the impairment of mitochondrial cristae affecting cardiac morphology and function is induced by pressure overload [44].

3.3 Regulation of autophagy in the heart

Excessive caloric intake results in obesity, a major independent risk factor for cardiovascular disease, including cardiac hypertrophy and heart failure. From this standpoint, cardiac remodeling is modulated by overnutrition or starvation. The adipokine leptin mediates energy balance between adipose tissue and the brain. Leptin and its receptors (LepRs) are expressed in the heart. LepRs belong to the class I cytokine receptor family signaling via JAK (Janus kinase)-2 and signal transducer and activator of transcription (STAT)-3. In addition, nutrient signaling mediators, such as mTOR (mammalian target of rapamycin), induce LepR-mediated activation of Akt. Cellular hypertrophy, proliferation and survival play an important role in cardiovascular function and pathology mediated by the Akt/mTOR pathway [45]. To examine the importance of endothelial leptin signaling in cardiac hypertrophy, transverse aortic constriction was used in mice with inducible endothelium-specific deletion of leptin receptors (End.LepR-KO) or littermate controls (End.LepR-WT). Histology and quantitative polymerase chain reaction analysis confirmed reduced cardiomyocyte hypertrophy. STAT3 activation was reduced, and Akt (protein kinase B) and mTOR phosphorylation after transverse aortic constriction were blunted in End.LepR-KO mice hearts [46].

For normal cardiac physiology in response to pressure overload (PO), mTORC2 is also required to ensure cardiomyocyte survival. It has been observed that dysregulation of autophagy in cardiomyocytes is implicated in various heart disease conditions. In these cases, vigorous protein quality control (PQC) systems are essential for maintaining the long-term well-being of nonproliferating mammalian cells, such as neurons and cardiomyocytes (CMs) [47]. Similarly, PO activates autophagy in at least an acute phase and the suppression of PO-induced autophagy that alleviates pathological cardiac remodeling. Recent investigations revealed that enhancing autophagy ameliorates desmin-related cardiomyopathies, which are inherited cardiomyopathies that result in severe heart failure due to protein aggregation and myofibrillar disarray in CMs [47].

3.4 New therapeutic objective of metabolic cardiomyopathy in autophagy

Perturbations in autophagy are involved in virtually all stages of cardiovascular disease. Research in the last decade has revealed that autophagy in cardiomyocytes plays a protective role, but not only during hemodynamic stress, but also in homeostasis during aging, resulting in mitochondrial damage. These damaged mitochondria are degraded through mitophagy and this process could be the main protective function of autophagy in the heart. From this standpoint, the mTORC1 complex regulates numerous biological processes, including proliferation, protein synthesis and autophagy inhibition. In addition, the mTORC1 pathway inhibits phosphorylation of the ULK1 protein (Ser 757) [48] considered an important element of autophagy activation.

The effects of mTOR are mediated through its activity as a central inhibitor of autophagy, a highly conserved cellular survival mechanism by which nutrient-deprived cells refresh the bioavailability of metabolic precursors [6]. In the cardiovascular system, the mTOR pathway regulates the physiological and pathological processes in the heart. In this regard, mTORC2 is necessary to maintain normal cardiac physiology and it ensures the survival of cardiomyocytes that have been subjected to PO. However, partial genetic or pharmacological inhibition of mTORC1 has been shown to reduce cardiac remodeling and heart failure in response to PO and chronic myocardial infarction. Therefore, mTOR may be a therapeutic strategy to confer cardioprotection [45].

Nonetheless, depending on the context, autophagic flux may be biased up or down. A large body of preclinical evidence suggests that autophagy is a double-edged sword in cardiovascular disease, acting in either beneficial or maladaptive ways, depending on the context. Modulation of Beclin 1 significantly influences both autophagy and apoptosis, thereby deeply affecting the survival and death of cardiomyocytes in the heart. This is the reason why it is important to discuss the signaling mechanism of autophagy modulation through Beclin 1, including the therapeutic potential of Beclin 1 in heart diseases [49]. In light of this, the autophagic machinery in cardiomyocytes and other cardiovascular cell types has been proposed as potential therapeutic targets. Autophagy mediators hold promise as targets for cardiovascular disease therapy; however, recent evidence suggesting that titration of autophagic flux holds potential as a new therapeutic goal for cardiovascular diseases, and heart failure, needs to be analyzed further [40].

3.5 Treatment for autophagy

The use of pharmacological modulators can be beneficial for the treatment and prevention of autophagy. It is known that many agents or procedures induce or reduce autophagy activity; among these are spermidine, carvedilol, trehalose, resveratrol, metformin, caloric restriction, exercise training, intermittent fasting and ischemia/reperfusion.

Fasting and calorie restriction are the most potent nongenetic autophagy stimulators related to autophagy promotion. Regarding the upregulation of autophagy, the evidence overwhelmingly suggests that autophagy has to be induced in a wide variety of tissues and organs in response to food deprivation. From a mechanistic point of view, age-related vascular remodeling is driven by a greater accumulation of ROS. Thus, the induction of autophagy per se is sufficient to extend the shelf life in various species ranging from yeast to mammals [50]. Therefore, in addition to preserving the homeostasis of organisms in baseline physiological conditions, autophagy also contributes to metabolic fitness and the adaptation to stressful conditions, such as nutrient deprivation, hypoxia, OS or physical exercise.

Autophagy is a critical process for cell homeostasis and survival, and it is also implicated in the reduction of OS and inflammation. Furthermore, autophagic processes have been associated with a greater expression of eNOS and bioavailability of the protein. Long-lived, damaged, dysfunctional and potentially harmful cellular components break down for detoxification, energy production and cell renewal, providing building components and stimulating anabolic processes for effective cell recycling.

Vascular induction of NO production as a response to shear stress during exercise with augmented blood flow and increased flux sanguin over endothelial cells (EC) result in eNOS activation and NO production. Autophagic process has been related to greater expression of eNOS and bioavailability of the protein. ATG3 is an important autophagy pathway mediator; in contrast with a reduction of 85% by knockdown of ATG3 protein expression using control siRNA upon exposure to shear stress showed impairment of eNOS activation and as a result were incapable of produce NO as a response to shear stress. Autophagy is a critical process for cell homeostasis and survival is also implicated. Long-lived, damaged, dysfunctional and potentially harmful cellular components break down for detoxification, energy production and cell renewal, providing building components and stimulating anabolic processes for effective cell recycling as a result of autophagy [51].

3.5.1 Exercise-mediated regulation of autophagy

Substantial evidence indicates that exercise training plays a beneficial role in the prevention and treatment of CV diseases. The regulation of autophagy during exercise is a bidirectional process. Autophagy is a physiologic process that is a defense mechanism for cells in adverse environments and it is also involved in several pathological processes [52]. Autophagy normal levels confer cell protection versus environmental stimuli to balance and protect organisms [53]. In this context, various diseases are the response to excessive or insufficient autophagy. Exercise training, referring generally to the cardiac adaptation to exercise, which has to be in an appropriate intensity as a chronic stimulation process, can reduce the risk of CV diseases and improve the prognosis of patients after CV events. This type of training can also reduce the production of ROS, reduce the inflammatory response, regulate collagen metabolism, moderate the imbalance of extracellular matrix synthesis and degradation, and alleviate cardiac fibrosis [54].

3.5.2 Intermittent fasting

Calorie restriction and stimulation of autophagy have healthy effects on the lifespan and cardioprotection in humans. Intermittent fasting induces adverse ventricular remodeling and cardiomyocyte death in null mice with LAMP2 (lysosome-associated membrane protein 2) associated with an impaired autophagic flow. The study of Godar et al. [54] highlights that intermittent fasting conferred cardioprotection in wild-type female mice, with an ~50% reduction in infarct size compared to controls matched without fasting, and this cardioprotection was lost in heterozygous null mice for LAMP2. One of the characteristics of these heterozygous null mice is the accumulation of damaged mitochondria with a deteriorated basal autophagic flux even on a fed day fed after 6 weeks, which probably results in the loss of cardioprotection observed with this regimen in wild-type mice. Intermittent fasting modulates OS from the myocardium through the effects on the mitochondria, where it is lost in the context of LAMP2 ablation due to the deterioration of mitochondrial autophagy [55]. Recent studies have discovered a potential mechanism for transcriptional replacement of autophagy-lysosome machinery with starvation. In addition, a central role was attributed to dephosphorylation and the cytoplasm induced by rapid hunger to nuclear translocation of TFEB (EB transcription factor) [55]. The endogenous TFEB-mediated stimulation of the autophagic flow is essential for the cytoprotective effects of repetitive hunger in hypoxia-reoxygenation injury. The research group suggests the hypothesis that the transcriptional replenishment of the autophagy-lysosome machinery by fasting (and hunger as described earlier) may be a critical determinant of beneficial autophagy, which allows living organisms to survive in what has probably been one of the first evolutionary stresses that accompanied the origin of life [56].

Therefore, starvation (total caloric restriction) is a potent stimulus for the induction of myocardial macroautophagy (called "autophagy") [57–59]. It is already known that autophagy is essential for cardiac homeostasis in the period of perinatal hunger at birth; this effect is observed before the establishment of breast milk supply [60]. In experiments using mice with genetic ablation of autophagy proteins ATG5 and ATG7, autophagosomes could not be formed and fatal myocardial ischemia developed [60, 61]. In this respect, autophagy is also essential for the maintenance of cardiac structure and function during prolonged starvation in mice, since the concomitant deterioration of autophagy with FOXo1 genetic ablation, Becn1 haplo-insufficiency [57] or pharmacological inhibition with bafilomycin A1 [62], an inhibitor of acidification and lysosome function, produces a rapid development of cardiomyopathy with starvation.

3.5.3 Ischemia/reperfusion

The different roles of autophagy in cardiomyocytes exposed to varying degrees of ischemia/reperfusion injury (I/R) or severe anoxia (S/A) were explored, and it was observed that the autophagic activity of cardiomyocytes increased with an increment in ischemia that was dependent on the duration of anoxia, undergoing ischemia, or severe ischemia [63].

During the process of cardiac ischemia, the restriction in the blood supply and the reduction of ATP leads to an imbalance in the amount of blood and energy, causing cell heart dysfunction and myocardial damage, inflammation and excess of ROS production leading to cardiomyocyte death. It should be noted that ATP levels can be monitored by adenosine monophosphate-activated protein kinase (AMPK), which functions as a nutrient deprivation sensor in response to a decreased ATP level during cardiac ischemia [64].

In the initial phase of ischemia, a low level of ATP activates AMPK in cardiomyocytes. Once activated, AMPK directly phosphorylates and activates ULK1 resulting in the induction of autophagy by modifying ULK1 directly or indirectly [48]. The pathway by which AMPK activates autophagy is through AMPK/mTORC1 signaling. AMPK inhibits mTORC1 through phosphorylation of TSC2 and the raptor site, followed by indirect activation of ULK1 [48]. Recent studies revealed new pathways through which AMPK activated autophagy. Also, AMPK directly phosphorylates and activates activated ULK1, allowing the onset of autophagy [65–67]. Also, in the early I/R process, ROS modify the function of Ca^{2+} channels and exchangers, which triggers a decrease in available ATP, and thus, directly affect the autophagy process [68].

Beclin 1 is an important autophagic protein that has been shown to regulate both the formation and processing of autophagosomes, especially in the reperfusion phase. An in vitro study revealed that autophagic response to nutrient deprivation mediated by Beclin 1 is modulated by the Bcl-2 protein in cardiac cells [69]. Moreover, it has been observed that ROS can also be strong inducers of Beclin 1 in mediating autophagy during the reperfusion phase [70]. In addition to regulating Beclin 1 expression, ROS could also oxidize and decrease ATG4 activity, contributing to LC3 lipidation at the start of autophagy [71].

Cellular stress by ischemia, hypoxia, depletion of intracellular Ca^{2+} stores, induced OS and ROS, and the accumulation of unfolded/misfolded proteins induce ER dysfunction known as ER stress, and then the unfolded protein response (UPR) is generated to deal and play a critical role in cell death after myocardial I/R injury. Several transcription factors are induced by ER stress and the UPR whose branch includes ATF6, inositol-requiring enzyme 1 (IRE1) and PKR-like ER kinase (PERK) activated by I/R injury, which is the mediated signal pathway of UPR. The activating transcription factor 6 alpha (ATF6) is an ER transmembrane protein and most ATF6-induced proteins localize to the ER [72].

Catalase is an enzyme that has been shown to decrease damaging ROS in the heart. ATF6 induces catalase known to decrease ROS and reduce I/R damage in the heart. Catalase is a component of peroxisomes that has also been found in the cytosol and cardiac mitochondria, and it neutralizes H_2O_2 and also serves to oxidize ONOO—, NO and organic peroxides; however, it has not be found in the ER. In the study by Jin et al. [72], they examined the effects of blocking ATF6-induced proteins in the ER stress response on I/R injury in cardiac myocytes and mouse hearts. The role of ATF6 as a link between ER stress and OS and its effect on I/R myocardial injury show an important function for ATF6, which binds to specific elements in the regulatory elements of the catalase gene inducing its transcription [72].

Myocardial I/R injury negatively regulates protein synthesis, leading to the activation of signaling pathways from the ER to the cytosol and nucleus, representing UPR and ER-associated protein degradation (ERAD). Most of I/R damage is caused by ROS generated outside the ER. The study by Zhang et al. revealed that all the three branches of UPR pathway are involved. Moreover, they demonstrated reduced myocardium damage in I/R surgery, while the activation of UPR had opposite effects. The results of this study were shown after the inhibition using a standardized animal model with Sprague-Dawley rats that were pretreated with UPR stimulator dithiothreitol (DTT) and UPR inhibitor 4-phenylbutyrate (4PBA) and then subjected to myocardial I/R surgery [73].

Under the cardiac I/R condition, increased autophagic activity compensated for impaired UPS function, thereby maintaining proteolysis at an appropriate level. However, cooperation between UPS (short-lived proteins) and autophagy (long-lived proteins) is considered a housekeeping mechanism for protein quality control in I/R injury. Thus, this increased autophagic response helps to maintain an adequate proteolysis level and proteostasis in order to compensate impaired UPS function under cardiac I/R condition, which ultimately results in degradation by the proteasome as well as autophagy.

3.5.4 Spermidine

Spermidine (SPD) is a type of polyamine that has been shown to enhance heart function to delay cellular and organismal aging and provide cardiovascular protection in humans. Initially, the cardioprotective effects of SPD were explored in rodent models of physiological cardiac aging (mice) and congestive heart failure induced by high salt concentration (rats) [74]. SPD in the diet of mice delays cardiac aging by improving diastolic function.

Furthermore, the evidence demonstrated that a high intake of SPD in the diet was correlated with a reduction in the incidence of cardiovascular diseases. In humans, high levels of SPD (natural polyamine) in the diet, as assessed by food questionnaires, correlated with reduced blood pressure and a lower incidence of cardiovascular disease. Subsequently, SPD was identified as a potent inducer of autophagy [74]. SPD by increasing autophagic and mitophageal activity improves mitochondrial respiratory function. SPD also inhibited kidney damage and fibrosis. It is suggested that the effect of SPD on the improvement of cardiac function is mediated by the promotion of autophagy and mitophagy in the heart and by the reduction of the systemic chronic inflammatory response. This natural polyamine is importantly involved in maintaining cellular homeostasis, and it affects several processes including cell growth, proliferation and tissue regeneration; it also stimulates the antineoplastic immune response and anti-aging properties, including transcriptional and transductional modulation through several enzymes and nucleic acid enzymes. Moreover, SPD promotes chaperone activity and ensures proteostasis through anti-inflammatory and antioxidant properties, and it also enhances mitochondrial function and cellular respiration [75].

Therefore, the effect of exogenous SDP administration was examined in aged rat hearts [76]. SPD was shown to improve mitochondrial biogenesis by increasing nuclear expression of PGC-1α (peroxisome proliferator-activated receptor gamma coactivator alpha), which is mediated by enhanced NAD^+-dependent deacetylase activity of SIRT1 (sirtuin-1). These results suggest that SIRT1 is an essential intermediary in the mechanism by which SPD stimulates mitochondrial biogenesis and function in cardiac cells. In addition, findings showed that the administration of SPD in vivo increased the activity of the antioxidant enzymes, superoxide dismutase (SOD) and catalase (CAT), and improved mitochondrial respiratory activity in the myocardium [76]. To date, there are not enough clinical trials to evaluate the effects of SPD in reducing cardiovascular diseases. These findings could guide new therapeutic strategies to counteract cardiac aging and prevent age-related cardiovascular disease and, as a result, lay the foundation for better heart disease treatments related to mitochondrial dysfunction [76].

3.5.5 Carvedilol

Carvedilol (CVL) belongs to the so-called α, β blockers, used to treat high blood pressure and congestive heart failure, which are generally used for the treatment of cardiovascular disorders. CVL blocks sympathetic neural activation through antagonism of the β1, β2 and α1 adrenoceptors and it has demonstrated greater cardiovascular benefits than traditional β blockers in both humans and animals. However, some benefits beyond decreased blood pressure were observed clinically, suggesting the potential anti-inflammatory activity of CVL [77]. In addition, CVL is a known membrane "fluidizer" that alters membrane structure and protein-lipid interactions [78]. The most widely characterized inflammasome sensor in the heart is activated in response to noninfectious stimuli, such as cell debris during acute myocardial infarction. The NOD-like receptor (NLR) family, pyrin domain–containing protein 3 (NLRP3) inflammasome is a component of the inflammatory process. Activation of the NLRP3 inflammasome triggers further myocardial damage indirectly through the release of IL-1β and directly through the promotion of inflammatory cell death via pyroptosis [79]. Pyroptosis is a type of caspase-1–dependent cell death, which is often associated with inflammasome activation and IL-1β production characterized by a loss of cell membrane integrity that leads to fluid influx and cell swelling [77]. Experimental studies have shown that strategies inhibiting the activation of the NLRP3 inflammasome in the early reperfusion period after acute myocardial infarction reduce the overall size of the infarct and preserve normal cardiac function [79]. There is also evidence supporting the therapeutic value of NLRP3 inflammasome-targeted strategies in experimental models and data supporting the role of the NLRP3 inflammasome in AMI and its consequences on adverse cardiac remodeling, cytokine-mediated systolic dysfunction and heart failure [79]. Mechanistic analysis revealed that CVL prevented lysosomal and mitochondrial damage and reduced apoptosis-associated speck-like protein containing a CARD (ASC) oligomerization. Additionally, CVL caused autophagic induction through a SIRT1-dependent pathway, which inhibited the NLRP3 inflammasome [77].

CVL activates survival signaling of p-AKT and pluripotential markers in cardiomyocytes (CM) after I/R. Cardioprotective actions of CVL are associated with higher levels of the miR-199a-3p and miR-214 cardioprotective miRNAs [79]. CVL stimulates the processing of microRNA (MIR)-199a-3p and miR-214 in the heart through β-arrestin-1–biased β-1 adrenergic receptor (β1 AR) for cardioprotective signaling. Studies show that using cultured cardiomyocyte and primary cardiomyocyte cell lines, carvedilol is regulated by an increase in miR-199a-3p and miR-214 in ventricular and atrial cardiomyocytes undergoing reperfusion ischemia (I/R) injury.

3.5.6 Trehalose

It is known that trehalose, a natural disaccharide, protects cells against various stresses. Trehalose is a natural disaccharide formed from two glucose molecules with an α-type glycosidic junction. It is widely distributed in nonmammalian species, such as fungi, yeasts, bacteria, invertebrates, insects and plants. Trehalose acts to provide energy sources and protect the integrity of cells exposed to various environmental stresses. Furthermore, it has also been shown that trehalose protects against apoptosis in an autophagy-dependent manner. This natural disaccharide improves cardiac remodeling, fibrosis and apoptosis after myocardial infarction and attenuated heart dysfunction [80]. The cardioprotective effect of trehalose was not observed in the heterozygous elimination of Beclin 1 in mice, indicating that these protective effects are mediated by autophagy [81]. In this connection, trehalose induces autophagy by facilitating the recruitment of LC3B to the autophagosomal membranes in an mTOR-independent manner. The basal level of autophagy plays a unique housekeeping role in the regulation of cardiac geometry and impaired autophagy function and may contribute to various end-organ complications in insulin resistance and diabetes, including cardiomyopathy and nephropathy [82]. Autophagy is usually regulated by both mTOR-dependent and -independent mechanisms. The mTOR pathway is considered the classic autophagy regulation route, which negatively regulates autophagy involving two functional complexes: mTORC1 and mTORC2, with a much more predominant role for mTORC1. Research findings suggest that trehalose may rescue the contractile myocardial defect induced by insulin resistance and apoptosis, through autophagy associated with the dephosphorylation of p38 MAPK and FOXo1 without affecting the phosphorylation of Akt [82]. Moreover, it was observed that trehalose not only activated autophagy but also increased the expression of p62. In addition, the expression of antioxidant genes regulated by trehalose through enhanced nuclear translocation of Nrf2 in a p62-dependent manner leads to the suppression of OS. Therefore, a new antioxidant action target for trehalose was proposed [83].

3.5.7 Lysosomal inhibitors blocking autophagy

Several lysosomal inhibitors such as bafilomycin A1 (BafA1), protease inhibitors and chloroquine (CQ) have been used interchangeably to block autophagy in vitro for lysosomal degradation. Only CQ and its derivate hydroxychloroquine (HCQ) are FDA-approved drugs currently considered the principal compounds used in clinical trials aimed for treating tumors through autophagy inhibition by impairing autophagosome fusion [84]. They focus on how CQ inhibits autophagy and directly compare its effects to those of BafA1. CQ mainly inhibits autophagy by impairing autophagosome fusion with lysosomes rather than by affecting the acidity and/or degradative activity of this organelle. Furthermore, CQ induces an autophagy-independent severe disorganization of the Golgi and endolysosomal systems, which impair autophagosome fusion. These results of Mauthe et al. suggest not using these compounds (CQ and HCQ) for in vivo experiments because of multiple cellular alterations caused by these drugs [84].

3.5.8 Resveratrol

Human clinical studies differ markedly in terms of the administered doses of resveratrol, as well as in the duration of treatment. Overall, the most pronounced effects of resveratrol include reduced body weight in obese patients and a partial decrease in systolic blood pressure, as well as fasting blood glucose levels and HbA1c in patients with diabetes mellitus in some clinical trials. Studies show that resveratrol attenuates high glucose-induced cardiomyocyte apoptosis through AMPK, a serine/threonine kinase that detects the state of cellular energy and regulates energy homeostasis [85]. Activation of AMPK is involved in the determination of multiple cellular processes including cell growth, apoptosis [86] and autophagy [87]. It is known that AMPK activation could inhibit mTOR, the best characterized protein kinase that negatively regulates autophagy [88]. Diabetic cardiomyopathy has shown inhibition of autophagy and increased apoptosis in cardiac cells. The study of Xu et al. demonstrated that using resveratrol in H9c2 cardiac myoblast cells exposed to high glucose combined with palmitate suppressed autophagic activity and increased apoptotic cell death. The H9c2 cells showed restored autophagy and attenuated apoptosis in cells with diabetic stimuli when treated with resveratrol [89, 90].

3.5.9 Metformin

Metformin is a first-line antidiabetic drug that also activates autophagy and it has cardiovascular protective effects [91], although a recent study reported otherwise, since metformin did not achieve the cardioprotective effect in an I/R model in nonaged pigs [92]. This was proven because the protective effect of metformin was abolished by treatment with chloroquine. This treatment inhibits the fusion of lysosomes with autophagosomes and a high lysosomal pH, avoids the final digestion stage and inhibits lysosomal activity [93].

However, a recent study by Chen Li et al. showed protection with metformin on both cellular and animal models of aging and I/R injury. During aging, failure of organelles results in the accumulation of macromolecules and impaired proteostasis that result in the death of cardiac tissue. Necroptosis is a programmed cell death involving receptor-interacting protein kinases 1 and 3 (RIP1, RIP3) that form the necrosome and mixed lineage kinase domain-like protein (MLKL), which are subsequently phosphorylated [94]. Besides, metformin treatment was able to restore autophagy and reduce the accumulation of p62 in the aged myocardium, as well as decrease the cardiac junction of p62-RIP1-RIP3 complexes and the RIP3 and MLKL-induced phosphorylation. Therefore, metformin can break the unfavorable chain mechanism of aging-related autophagy decrease that induces necroptosis [94].

3.6 Development of new autophagy modulators

Diabetes is a metabolic disorder that contributes to the development of cardiac fibrosis and cardiomyopathy. Aminoguanidine (AG) inhibits advanced glycation end products (AGEs) and advanced oxidation protein products (AOPP) accumulated as a result of excessive oxidative stress in diabetes. In a recent work, we investigated whether AG supplementation mitigates oxidative-associated cardiac fibrosis in rats with type 2 diabetes mellitus (T2DM). In vivo experiments were performed in a model of T2DM, and in vitro we used primary rat myofibroblasts to confirm the antioxidant and antifibrotic effects of AG to determine if blocking the receptor for AGEs (RAGE) prevents the fibrogenic response in myofibroblasts. Diabetic rats exhibited an increase in cardiac fibrosis resulting from a high-fat, high-carbohydrate diet (HFCD) and streptozotocin (STZ) injections. In contrast, AG treatment significantly reduced cardiac fibrosis, alfa-smooth muscle actin (αSMA) and oxidative-associated NOX4 and NOS2 mRNA expression [95]. In vitro challenge of myofibroblasts with AG under T2DM conditions reduced intra- and extracellular collagen type I expression and platelet-derived growth factor (PDGF), transforming growth factor beta (TGFβ1) and collagen type 1 a 1 (COL1A1) mRNAs, albeit with a similar expression of tumor necrosis factor alpha (TNFα) and interleukin-6 (IL-6) mRNAs. This was accompanied by reduced phosphorylation of extracellular signal-regulated kinase 1/2 (ERK1/2) and SMAD2/3 but not of AKT1/2/3 and signal transducer and activator of transcription (STAT) pathways. RAGE blockade further attenuated collagen type I expression in AG-treated myofibroblasts. Thus, AG reduces oxidative stress-associated cardiac fibrosis by reducing pERK1/2, pSMAD2/3 and collagen type I expression via AGE/RAGE signaling in T2DM [95]. However, clinical studies need to be performed in order to evaluate if AG treatment is useful and well-tolerated in human cardiac disease and leads to a significant reduction in cardiac fibrosis as well as it modulates the expression of oxidative and fibrogenic response in myofibroblasts like in this disease model.

Although the autophagy modulators described above have great potential, there are currently no interventions aimed at modulating autophagy for human use. Despite this, there are already licensed medicines for use in humans, which activate or inhibit autophagy, such as rapamycin, chloroquine and HCQ, among others, that were not developed for this purpose [96]. The main clinical obstacle is that they have low pharmacological specificity for their objective, which is the autophagic

Increase AMPK		Decrease mTORC1
Caloric restriction Physical exercise H_2S Metformin Simvastatin A-769662	Initiation	Caloric restriction Physical exercise Everolimus Rapamycin Temsirolimus Torins
Increase ROS		Increase nuclear RF-1 Activation of MAPK
Antimycobacterial antibiotics Carbon monoxide Melatonin	Pre-phagophore induction	IFNγ
Increase MAPK		Inositol 1,4,5-triphosphate receptor
Carbamazepine Lithium	Nucleation	BECN1 activating peptide
Chromosome maintenance region-1 (CRM-1)		
Hydroxycitrate Resveratrol Spermidine	Elongation	
		Unknown
	Fusion	Chloramphenicol Retinoic acid
Unknown		
Trehalose Trichostatin A	Degradation	

Examples of autophagy activators. A-769662, a new activator of AMP-activated protein kinase (AMPK); BECN1, Beclin 1; H_2S, hydrogen sulfide; mTORC1, target of rapamycin complex 1.

Table 1.
Autophageal processes susceptible to therapeutic modulation.

process [84]. However, they have allowed us to know the main pathways by which the autophagy process is activated or inactivated. Several pharmacological and nutritional interventions are available to inhibit autophagy in the initiation, nucleation, elongation, fusion or degradation phase [97]. In addition, several agents modulate autophagy through multiple molecular mechanisms that are not yet characterized (**Table 1**).

4. Conclusions

Alteration of proteostasis in heart tissue leads to diabetic cardiomyopathy characterized by myocardial remodeling and interstitial fibrosis. Cardiomyocyte proteotoxicity frequently faces the chronic accumulation of misfolded or unfolded proteins that can lead to proteotoxic formation or aggregation of soluble peptides with reduced cardiac function and arrhythmias. However, under pathological conditions, autophagic flux may be an important strategy to prevent the progression of various cardiovascular diseases due to risk of dysfunctional endothelial cells. Autophagy is insufficient in endothelial cells isolated from individuals with diabetes mellitus. Moreover, it has been demonstrated that intact autophagy is essential for eNOS signaling in endothelial cells. Nitric oxide-mediated vasodilation was promoted by the induction of autophagy.

Autophagy has been shown to be a mechanism of fibrosis recovery and scarring secondary to cell apoptosis and active in the perimeter of cardiovascular fibrotic tissue. Autophagy inhibition has a beneficial effect on type 2 diabetes–induced cardiomyopathy. These findings suggest that autophagy is diversely altered in different types of diabetes-induced cardiac pathologies. Therefore, targeting autophagy regulation may be a potential therapeutic strategy for diabetic cardiomyopathy.

Moreover, the animal model of T2DM induced by STZ plus HFCD whose diabetic response evokes pro-oxidative and profibrotic attenuated reactions in the presence of AG suggests that this molecule may be part of autophagy therapy for diabetic cardiomyopathy. Thus, AG reduces oxidative stress-associated cardiac fibrosis by decreasing pERK1/2, pSMAD2/3 and collagen type I expression via AGE/RAGE signaling in T2DM.

The knowledge of the molecules involved in mechanisms of proteostasis and autophagy in cardiac cells and the role they play in various signaling pathways will serve as an opportunity for the future design of therapeutic targets for the treatment of fibrosis, alterations of cardiac tissue remodeling and cardiomyopathy.

Acknowledgements

This work was partially supported by grant from the academic group, SEP/PRODEP and CONACYT/PRO-SNI.

Conflict of interest

The authors declare no conflict of interest.

Author details

María Cristina Islas-Carbajal[1]*, Ana Rosa Rincón-Sánchez[2], Cesar Arturo Nava-Valdivia[3] and Claudia Lisette Charles-Niño[3]

1 Department of Physiology, Institute of Experimental and Clinical Therapeutics, University Center of Health Sciences, Guadalajara University, Guadalajara, Jalisco, Mexico

2 Department of Molecular Biology and Genomics, Institute of Molecular Biology and Gene Therapy, University Center of Health Sciences, Guadalajara University, Guadalajara, Jalisco, Mexico

3 Department of Microbiology and Pathology, University Center of Health Sciences, Guadalajara University, Guadalajara, Jalisco, Mexico

*Address all correspondence to: islascarbajal@yahoo.com; cristina.islas@academicos.udg.mx

References

[1] Guertl B, Noehammer C, Hoefler G. Metabolic cardiomyopathies. International Journal of Experimental Pathology. Dec 2000;**81**(6):349-372. DOI: 10.1046/j.1365-2613.200.00186.x

[2] Woodall BP, Gustafsson ÅB. Autophagy—A key pathway for cardiac health and longevity. Acta Physiologica (Oxford, England). 2018;**223**(4):e13074. DOI: 10.1111/apha.13074

[3] Abdellatif M, Sedej S, Carmona-Gutierrez D, Madeo F, Kroemer G. Autophagy in cardiovascular aging. Circulation Research. 2018;**123**:803-824. DOI: 10.1161/CIRCRESAHA.118.312208

[4] Hipp MS, Kasturi P, Ulrich Hartl F. The proteostasis network and its decline in ageing. Nature Reviews. Molecular Cell Biology. 2019;**20**:421-435. DOI: 10.1038/s41580-019-0101-y

[5] Alshehri AM. Metabolic syndrome and cardiovascular risk. Journal of Family & Community Medicine. 2010;**17**(2):73-78. DOI: 10.4103/1319-1683.71987

[6] Gogiraju R, Bochenek ML, Schäfer K. Angiogenic endothelial cell signaling in cardiac hypertrophy and heart failure. Frontiers in Cardiovascular Medicine. 2019;**6**(20):1-21. DOI: 10.3389/fcvm.2019.00020

[7] Ravid T, Hochstrasser M. Degradation signal diversity in the ubiquitin-proteasome system. Nature Reviews. Molecular Cell Biology. 2008;**9**(9):679-690. DOI: 10.1038/nrm2468

[8] Wade Harper J, Bennett EJ. Proteome complexity and the forces that drive proteome imbalance. Nature. 2016;**537**(7620):328-338. DOI: 10.1038/nature19947

[9] Hipp MS, Park S-H, Hartl FU. Proteostasis impairment in protein-misfolding and -aggregation diseases. Trends in Cell Biology. 2014;**24**(9):506-514. DOI: 10.1016/j.tcb.2014.05.003

[10] Hetz C, Chevet E, Oakes SA. Proteostasis control by the unfolded protein response. Nature Cell Biology. 2015;**17**:829-838

[11] Niforou K, Cheimonidou C, Trougakos IP. Molecular chaperones and proteostasis regulation during redox imbalance. Redox Biology. 2014;**2**:323-332

[12] Vilchez D, Simic MS, Dillin A. Proteostasis and aging of stem cells. Trends in Cell Biology. 2014;**24**:161-170

[13] Tanaka K, Matsuda N. Proteostasis and neurodegeneration: The roles of proteasomal degradation and autophagy. Biochimica et Biophysica Acta - Molecular Cell Research. 2014;**1843**:197-204. Available from: http://www.ncbi.nlm.nih.gov/pubmed/23523933

[14] Soares TR, Reis SD, Pinho BR, Duchen MR, Oliveira JMA. Targeting the proteostasis network in Huntington's disease. Ageing Research Reviews. 2019;**49**:92-103

[15] Balch WE, Morimoto RI, Dillin A, Kelly JW. Adapting proteostasis for disease intervention. Science. 2008;**319**:916-919. DOI: 10.1126/science.1141448

[16] Ravanan P, Srikumar IF, Talwar P. Autophagy: The spotlight for cellular stress responses. Life Sciences. 2017;**188**:53-67. DOI: 10.1016/j.lfs.2017.08.029

[17] Finley D. Recognition and processing of ubiquitin-protein conjugates by the proteasome. Annual Review of Biochemistry. 2009;**78**(1):477-513. DOI: 10.1146/annurev.biochem.78.081507.101607

[18] Massey AC, Kiffin R, Cuervo AM. Autophagic defects in aging: Looking for

an "emergency exit"? Cell Cycle. 2006;**5**: 1292-1296

[19] Kobayashi S, Liang Q. Autophagy and mitophagy in diabetic cardiomyopathy. Biochimica et Biophysica Acta (BBA): Molecular Basis of Disease. 2015;**1852**(2):252-261

[20] Wang X, Su H, Ranek MJ, et al. Protein quality control and degradation in cardiomyocytes. Journal of Molecular and Cellular Cardiology. 2008;**45**:11-27

[21] Melkani GC, Bhide S, Han A, et al. TRiC/CCT chaperonins are essential for maintaining myofibril organization, cardiac physiological rhythm, and lifespan. FEBS Letters. 2017;**591**: 3447-3458

[22] Taneike M, Yamaguchi O, Nakai A, et al. Inhibition of autophagy in the heart induces age-related cardiomyopathy. Autophagy. 2010;**6**: 600-606

[23] Tania Zaglia G, Milan A, Ruhs M, Franzoso E, Bertaggia N, Pianca A, et al. Atrogin-1 deficiency promotes cardiomyopathy and premature death via impaired autophagy. The Journal of Clinical Investigation. 2014;**124**(6): 2410-2424. DOI: 10.1172/JCI66339

[24] Massague J. TGF-beta signalling in context. Nature Reviews. Molecular Cell Biology. 2012;**13**:616-630

[25] He C, Klionsky DJ. Regulation mechanisms and signaling pathways of autophagy. Annual Review of Genetics. 2009;**43**:67-93

[26] Ghavami S, Cunnington RH, Gupta S, et al. Autophagy is a regulator of TGF-β1-induced fibrogenesis in primary human atrial myofibroblasts. Cell Death & Disease. 2015;**6**:1696

[27] Jalil JE, Doering CW, Janicki JS, et al. Fibrillar collagen and myocardial stiffness in the intact hypertrophied rat left ventricle. Circulation Research. 1989;**64**:1041-1050

[28] Kim G, Jun JB, Elkon KB. Necessary role of phosphatidylinositol 3-kinase in transforming growth factor beta-mediated activation of Akt in normal and rheumatoid arthritis synovial fibroblasts. Arthritis and Rheumatism. 2002;**46**:1504-1511

[29] Stacchiotti A, Bonomini F, Lavazza A, et al. Adverse effects of cyclosporine a on HSP25, alpha B-crystallin and myofibrillar cytoskeleton in rat heart. Toxicology. 2009;**262**(3):192-198

[30] Kubli DA, Cortez MQ, Moyzis AG, et al. PINK1 is dispensable for mitochondrial recruitment of Parkin and activation of mitophagy in cardiac myocytes. PLoS One. 2015;**10**(6): 0130707

[31] Whelan RS, Kaplinskiy V, Kitsis RN. Cell death in the pathogenesis of heart disease: Mechanisms and significance. Annual Review of Physiology. 2010;**72**: 19-44

[32] Kanamori H, Takemura G, Goto K, et al. The role of autophagy emerging in postinfarction cardiac remodelling. Cardiovascular Research. 2011;**91**: 330-339

[33] Xiao Y, Wu QQ, Duan MX, Liu C, Yuan Y, Yang Z, et al. TAX1BP1 overexpression attenuates cardiac dysfunction and remodeling in STZ-induced diabetic cardiomyopathy in mice by regulating autophagy. Biochimica et Biophysica Acta (BBA): Molecular Basis of Disease. 2018;**1864**:1728-1743. DOI: 10.1016/j.bbadis.2018.02.012

[34] Förstermann U, Li H. Therapeutic effect of enhancing endothelial nitric oxide synthase (eNOS) expression and preventing eNOS uncoupling. British Journal of Pharmacology. 2011;**164**(2): 213-223. DOI: 10.1111/j.1476-5381.2010.01196.x

[35] Quan Y, Xin Y, Geer Tian G, Zhou J, Liu X. Mitochondrial oxidative stress and energy metabolism: Impact on aging and longevity. Hindawi Oxidative Medicine and Cellular Longevity. 2020:11. DOI: 10.1155/2020/9423593. Article ID 9423593

[36] Klionsky DJ, Abdelmohsen K, Abe A, Abedin MJ, Abeliovich H, Acevedo Arozena A, et al. Guidelines for the use and interpretation of assays for monitoring autophagy (3rd edition). Autophagy. 2016;**12**:1-222. DOI: 10.1080/15548627.2015.1100356.

[37] Li J, Zhang D, Wiersma M, Brundel BJJM. Role of autophagy in proteostasis: Friend and foe in cardiac diseases. Cell. 2018;7:279

[38] Denton D, Xu T, Kumar S. Autophagy as a pro-death pathway. Immunology & Cell Biology. 2015; **93**(1):35-42

[39] Kundu M, Thompson CB. Autophagy: Basic principles and relevance to disease. Annual Review of Pathology: Mechanisms of Disease. 2008;**3**:427-455. DOI: 10.1146/annurev.pathmechdis.2.010506.091842

[40] Schiattarella GG, Hill JA. Therapeutic targeting of autophagy in cardiovascular disease. Journal of Molecular and Cellular Cardiology. 2016;**95**:86-93. DOI: 10.1016/j.yjmcc.2015.11.019.

[41] Yamaguchi O. Autophagy in the heart. Circulation. 2019;**83**:697-704. DOI: 10.1253/circj.CJ-18-1065

[42] Nishida K, Otsu K. Autophagy during cardiac remodeling. Journal of Molecular and Cellular Cardiology. 2016;**95**:11-18

[43] Pedro JMB-S, Kroemer G, Galluzzi L. Autophagy and mitophagy in cardiovascular disease. Circulation Research. 2017;**120**:1812-1824. DOI: 10.1161/CIRCRESAHA.117.311082

[44] Oka T, Hikoso S, Yamaguchi O, Taneike M, Takeda T, Tamai T, et al. Mitochondrial DNA that escapes from autophagy causes inflammation and heart failure. Nature. 2012;**485**(7397): 251-255. DOI: 10.1038/nature10992

[45] Sciarretta S, Forte M, Frati G, Sadoshima J. New insights into the role of mTOR signaling in the cardiovascular system. Circulation Research. 2018;**122**: 489-505. DOI: 10.1161/CIRCRESAHA.117.311147

[46] Bagherniya M, Butler AE, Barreto GE, Sahebkar A. The effect of fasting or calorie restriction on autophagy induction: A review of the literature. Ageing Research Reviews. 2018;**47**:183-197. DOI: 10.1016/j.arr.2018.08.004

[47] Madeo F, Tavernarakis N, Kroemer G. Can autophagy promote longevity? Nature Cell Biology. 2010;**12**: 842-846. DOI: 10.1038/ncb0910-842

[48] Kim J, Kundu M, Viollet B, Guan KL. AMPK and mTOR regulate autophagy through direct phosphorylation of Ulk1. Nature Cell Biology. 2011;**13**(2):132-141. DOI: 10.1038/ncb2152

[49] Maejima Y, Isobe M, Sadoshima J. Regulation of autophagy by Beclin 1 in the heart. Journal of Molecular and Cellular Cardiology. 2016;**95**:19-25

[50] Pallauf K, Rimbach G. Autophagy, polyphenols and healthy ageing. Ageing Research Reviews. 2013; **12**(1):237-252. DOI: 10.1016/j.arr.2012.03.008

[51] Bharath LP, Mueller R, Li Y, Ruan T, Kunz D, Goodrich R, et al. Impairment of autophagy in endothelial cells prevents shear-stress-induced increases in nitric oxide bioavailability. Canadian Journal of Physiology and Pharmacology. 2014;**92**(7):605-612. DOI: 10.1139/cjpp-2014-0017

[52] Chung KW, Chung HY. The effects of calorie restriction on autophagy: Role on aging intervention. Nutrients. 2019; **11**(2923):1-18. DOI: 10.3390/nu11122923

[53] Wang L, Wang J, Cretoiu D, Li G, Xiao J. Exercise-mediated regulation of autophagy in the cardiovascular system. Journal of Sport and Health Science. 2019;**00**:1-8. DOI: 10.1016/j.jshs.2019.10.001

[54] Godar RJ, Ma X, Liu H, et al. Repetitive stimulation of autophagy-lysosome machinery by intermittent fasting preconditions the myocardium to ischemia-reperfusion injury. Autophagy. 2015;**11**(9):1537-1560. DOI: 10.1080/15548627.2015.1063768

[55] Martina JA, Chen Y, Gucek M, Puertollano R. MTORC1 functions as a transcriptional regulator of autophagy by preventing nuclear transport of TFEB. Autophagy. 2012;**8**:903-914. DOI: 10.4161/auto.19653

[56] Hariharan N, Maejima Y, Nakae J, Paik J, Depinho RA, Sadoshima J. Deacetylation of FoxO by Sirt1 plays an essential role in mediating starvation-induced autophagy in cardiac myocytes. Circulation Research. 2010;**107**: 1470-1482

[57] Mizushima N, Yamamoto A, Matsui M, Yoshimori T, Ohsumi Y. In vivo analysis of autophagy in response to nutrient starvation using transgenic mice expressing a fluorescent autophagosome marker. Molecular Biology of the Cell. 2004;**15**:1101-1111

[58] Zhu H, Tannous P, Johnstone JL, Kong Y, Shelton JM, Richardson JA, et al. Cardiac autophagy is a maladaptive response to hemodynamic stress. The Journal of Clinical Investigation. 2007;**117**:1782-1793

[59] Komatsu M, Waguri S, Ueno T, Iwata J, Murata S, Tanida I, et al. Impairment of starvation-induced and constitutive autophagy in Atg7-deficient mice. The Journal of Cell Biology. 2005; **169**:425-434. DOI: 10.1083/jcb.200412022

[60] Kuma A, Hatano M, Matsui M, Yamamoto A, Nakaya H, Yoshimori T, et al. The role of autophagy during the early neonatal starvation period. Nature. 2004;**432**:1032-1036. DOI: 10.1038/nature03029

[61] Kanamori H, Takemura G, Maruyama R, Goto K, Tsujimoto A, Ogino A, et al. Functional significance and morphological characterization of starvation-induced autophagy in the adult heart. The American Journal of Pathology. 2009;**174**:1705-1714. DOI: 10.2353/ajpath.2009.080875

[62] Xu Q, Li X, Lu Y, et al. Pharmacological modulation of autophagy to protect cardiomyocytes according to the time windows of ischaemia/reperfusion. British Journal of Pharmacology. 2015;**172**(12):3072-3085. DOI: 10.1111/bph.13111.

[63] Eisenberg T et al. Induction of autophagy by spermidine promotes longevity. Nature Cell Biology. 2009;**11**: 1305-1314

[64] Ma S, Wang Y, Chen Y, et al. The role of the autophagy in myocardial ischemia/reperfusion injury. Biochimica et Biophysica Acta (BBA): Molecular Basis of Disease. 2015; **1852**(2):271-276

[65] Egan D, Kim J, Shaw RJ, et al. The autophagy initiating kinase ULK1 is regulated via opposing phosphorylation by AMPK and mTOR. Autophagy. 2011; **7**:643-644

[66] Khan SH, Kumar R. Role of an intrinsically disordered conformation in AMPK-mediated phosphorylation of ULK1 and regulation of autophagy. Molecular BioSystems. 2012; **8**:91-96

[67] Alers S, Loffler AS, Wesselborg S, et al. Role of AMPK-mTOR-Ulk1/2 in the regulation of autophagy: Cross talk, shortcuts, and feedbacks. Molecular and Cellular Biology. 2012;**2**:2-1164

[68] Boulghobra D, Coste F, Geny B, et al. Exercise training protects the heart against ischemia-reperfusion injury: A central role for mitochondria? Free Radical Biology and Medicine. 2020;**152**: 395-410. DOI: 10.1016/j. freeradbiomed.2020.04.005

[69] Brady NR, Hamacher-Brady A, Yuan H, et al. The autophagic response to nutrient deprivation in the hl-1 cardiac myocyte is modulated by Bcl-2 and sarco/endoplasmic reticulum calcium stores. The FEBS Journal. 2007; **274**:3184-3197

[70] Hariharan N, Zhai P, Sadoshima J. Oxidative stress stimulates autophagic flux during ischemia/reperfusión. Antioxidants & Redox Signaling. 2011; **14**:2179-2190

[71] Scherz-Shouval R, Shvets E, Fass E, et al. Reactive oxygen species are essential for autophagy and specifically regulate the activity of Atg4. The EMBO Journal. 2007;**26**:1749-1760

[72] Jin J-K, Blackwood EA, Azizi K, Thuerauf DJ, Fahem AG, Hofmann C, et al. ATF6 decreases myocardial ischemia/reperfusion damage and links ER stress and oxidative stress signaling pathways in the heart. Circulation Research. 2017;**120**:862-875. DOI: 10.1161/CIRCRESAHA.116.310266

[73] Zhang C, Tang Y, Li Y, Xie L, Zhuang W, Liu J, et al. Unfolded protein response plays a critical role in heart damage after myocardial ischemia/ reperfusion in rats. PLoS One. 2017; **12**(6):e0179042. DOI: 10.1371/journal. pone.0179042

[74] Wang J, Li S, Wang J, Wu F, Yuhan C, Zhang H, et al. Spermidine alleviates cardiac aging by improving mitochondrial biogenesis and function. Aging. 2020;**12**(1):650-671. DOI: 10.18632/aging.102647

[75] Morselli E et al. Spermidine and resveratrol induce autophagy by distinct pathways converging on the acetylproteome. The Journal of Cell Biology. 2011;**192**:615-629

[76] Madeo F, Bauera MA, Carmona-Gutierreza D, Kroemer G. Spermidine: A physiological autophagy inducer acting as an anti-aging vitamin in humans? Autophagy. 2019;**15**(1):165-168. DOI: 10.1080/15548627.2018.1530929

[77] Wong WT, Li LH, Rao YK, et al. Reposicionamiento del bloqueador β Carvedilol Como un nuevo inductor de autofagia que inhibe el inflamatorio NLRP3. Frente Immunol. 2018;**9**:1920. DOI: 10.3389/fimmu.2018.01920

[78] Toldo S, Abbate A. The NLRP3 inflammasome in acute myocardial infarction. Nature Reviews. Cardiology. 2018;**15**:203-214

[79] Park KM, Teoh JP, Wang Y, et al. Carvedilol-responsive microRNAs, miR-199a-3p and -214 protect cardiomyocytes from simulated ischemia-reperfusion injury. American Journal of Physiology: Heart and Circulatory Physiology. 2016;**311**(2): H371-H383. DOI: 10.1152/ ajpheart.00807.2015

[80] Sciarretta S, Yee D, Nagarajan N, Bianchi F, Saito T, Valenti V, et al. Trehalose-induced activation of autophagy improves cardiac remodeling after myocardial infarction. Journal of the American College of Cardiology. 2018;**71**:1999-2010

[81] Wang Q, Ren J. mTOR–independent autophagy inducer trehalose rescues against insulin resistance –induced myocardial contractile anomalies: Role of p38

MAPK and Foxo 1. Pharmacological Research. 2016;**111**:357-373. DOI: 10.1016/j.phrs.2016.06.024

[82] Mizunoe Y, Kobayashi M, Sudo Y, et al. Trehalose protects against oxidative stress by regulating the Keap1-Nrf2 and autophagy pathways. Redox Biology. 2018;**15**:115-124. DOI: 10.1016/j.redox.2017.09.007.

[83] Madeo F, Zimmermann A, Maiuri MC, Kroemer G. Essential role for autophagy in life span extension. The Journal of Clinical Investigation. 2015;**125**(1):85-93. DOI: 10.1172/JCI73946

[84] Mauthe M, Orhon I, Rocchi C, Zhou X, Luhr M, Hijlkema K-J, et al. Chloroquine inhibits autophagic flux by decreasing autophagosome-lysosome fusion. Autophagy. 2018;**14**(8):1435-1455. DOI: 10.1080/15548627.2018.1474314

[85] Hardie DG. AMP-activated/SNF1 protein kinases: Conserved guardians of cellular energy. Nature Reviews. Molecular Cell Biology. 2007;**8**:774-785

[86] Shirwany NA, Zou MH. AMPK in cardiovascular health and disease. Acta Pharmacologica Sinica. 2010;**31**:1075-1084

[87] Herzig S, Shaw RJ. AMPK: Guardian of metabolism and mitochondrial homeostasis. Nature Reviews. Molecular Cell Biology. 2018;**19**:121-135

[88] Shaw RJ. LKB1 and AMP-activated protein kinase control of mTOR signalling and growth. Acta Physiologica (Oxf). 2009;**196**:65-80

[89] Mizushima N, Yoshimori T, Levine B. Methods in mammalian autophagy research. Cell. 2010;**140**:313-326

[90] Xu K, Liu XF, Ke ZQ, Yao Q, Guo S, Liu C. Resveratrol modulates apoptosis and autophagy induced by high glucose and palmitate in cardiac cells. Cellular Physiology and Biochemistry. 2018;**46**(5):2031-2040. DOI: 10.1159/000489442

[91] Song YM, Lee WK, Lee YH, Kang ES, Cha BS, Lee BW. Metformin restores Parkin-mediated mitophagy, suppressed by cytosolic p53. International Journal of Molecular Sciences. 2016;**17**(1):E122. DOI: 10.3390/ijms17010122

[92] Teng AC, Miyake T, Yokoe S, Zhang L, Rezende LM Jr, Sharma P, et al. Metformin increases degradation of phospholamban via autophagy in cardiomyocytes. Proceedings of the National Academy of Sciences of the United States of America. 2015;**112**(23):7165-7170. DOI: 10.1073/pnas.1508815112

[93] Techiryan G, Weil BR, Palka BA, Canty JM Jr. Effect of intracoronary metformin on myocardial infarct size in swine. Circulation Research. 2018;**123**(8):986-995. DOI: 10.1161/CIRCRESAHA.118.313341

[94] Davis JW, Ferro-Novick S. Crosstalk between the secretory and autophagy pathways regulates autophagosome formation. Developmental Cell. 2017;**41**:23-32. DOI: 10.1016/j.devcel.2017.03.015

[95] Magdaleno F, Blajszczak CC, Charles-Niño CL, Guadrón-Llanos AM, Vázquez-Álvarez AO, Miranda-Díaz AG, et al. Aminoguanidine reduces diabetes-associated cardiac fibrosis. Experimental and Therapeutic Medicine. 2019;**18**:3125-3138. DOI: 10.3892/etm.2019.7921

[96] Li C, Mu N, Gu C, et al. Metformin mediates cardioprotection against aging-induced ischemic necroptosis. Aging Cell. 2020;**19**(2):e13096. DOI: 10.1111/acel.13096

[97] Rubinsztein DC, Codogno P, Levine B. Autophagy modulation as a potential therapeutic target for diverse diseases. Nature Reviews. Drug Discovery. 2012;**11**(9):709-730. DOI: 10.1038/nrd3802

Section 2

Genetics of Vascular Pathologies

Chapter 4

Familial Hypercholesterolemia: Three "under" (Understood, Underdiagnosed, and Undertreated) Disease

Vladimir O. Konstantinov

Abstract

Familial hypercholesterolemia (FH) is one of the most prevalent genetic disorders leading to premature atherosclerosis and coronary heart disease. The main cause of FH is a mutation in the LDL-receptor gene that leads to loss of function of these receptors causing high levels of blood cholesterol. The diagnosis of FH is not very easy. Wide screenings are needed to reveal high levels of LDL cholesterol among "healthy" population. If the patient has MI or stroke at an early age, high levels of LDL cholesterol, and tendon xanthomas, the diagnosis of FH becomes much more clear. Genetic testing is a gold standard in the diagnosis of FH. There are several factors, influencing the time course of FH. Smoking males with low levels of HDL cholesterol have an extremely higher risk of death than nonsmoking females with high HDL cholesterol. Management of FH includes low cholesterol diet, statin and ezetimibe treatment, PCSK inhibitors, and LDL aphaeresis. Early and effective treatment influences much the prognosis in FH patients.

Keywords: prevalence of familial hypercholesterolemia (FH), diagnosis of FH, the time course of FH, treatment of FH

1. Introduction

Familial hypercholesterolemia (FH) is one of the most frequent inherited disorders caused mainly by a mutation of the gene encoding the low density lipoprotein receptor (LDLR). High concentrations of LDL result in uptake of LDL by extracellular matrix, including that of the arterial wall leading to premature atherosclerosis and coronary artery disease (CAD). CAD develops early with symptoms often manifesting in men in the fourth or fifth decade and women about 10 years later. Approximately 5% of all cases of premature myocardial infarction (MI) occur in patients with heterozygous FH [1, 2]. Before the development of statin therapy, at least 50% of FH male patients experienced MI by the age of 60. In homozygotes, symptomatic CAD can occur in childhood, and very few survive past the age of 30.

Brown and Goldstein are indisputably the fathers of FH. In 1972, they attributed the disorder to defective HMG-CoA reductase [3]. But, a year later they recognized that the main cause of the disease was the mutation in the LDLR gene [4]. The extremely rare homozygote with FH has two mutant alleles at the LDLR locus,

IntechOpen

leaving a person with an absolute or nearly absolute inability to clear LDL from circulation [1]. Brown and Goldstein initially described homozygous FH (HoFH) as a condition in which an individual inherits a single and same mutation in the LDLR from each parent. Now we recognize this condition as "simple HoFH" [5]. Actually, this is a very rare event. Far more frequently, HoFH is a result of inheritance of two different pathogenic mutations in the same gene that is referred to as a "compound heterozygote." Another type of HoFH is when an individual inherits a mutation of one gene (e.g., LDLR) from one of the parents and different gene (e.g., *apoB* or *PCSK9*) from another. This type of HoFH is a "double heterozygote." It is important to know that the term "heterozygote" is used here to describe homozygote patients.

Heterozygotes with FH possess one normal allele, giving them approximately one half of the normal receptor activity. Actually, LDLR also contributes to the clearance of VLDL remnants from the plasma, so a deficiency of LDLR may lead to some accumulation of remnant lipoproteins as well.

Additionally, mutations of other genes such as *apoB*, *PCSK9*, and so on are now recognized to also cause FH [6–8].

The prevalence of heterozygous FH (HeFH) is about 1/200 [9] and HoFH—1/160,000 [10, 11]. Therefore, HeFH is a very frequent disorder, and it is more common than type 1 diabetes mellitus. Unfortunately, the diagnosis of FH is often unrecognized, leaving such individuals and members of their families undertreated and of greater risk of consequences of lifelong LDL-C elevations. Nevertheless, the prevalence of FH may differ greatly in different populations. For example, in French Canadians, South African Afrikaners, Ashkenazi Jews, or Christian Lebanese, which are the so-called founder populations, the prevalence of FH can be as high as 1/67 [12, 13]. So, it is important to "know your audience" and be on the lookout for such individuals in daily clinical practice.

2. Discussion

The diagnosis of FH is simple and complicated at the same time. First of all patients with FH should have a very high LDL (>95% for age/gender matched controls) with typically normal TG and HDL. For patients with HoFH, LDL is >500 mg/dl (13 mmol/l) when untreated and >300 mg/dl (7.7 mmol/l)—on lipid-lowering therapy (LLT) [14–16]. The cut point for HeFH in adult had similarly been >190 mg/dl (5 mmol/l). Recent genotyping studies showed great difference in LDL levels among FH patients. To date, the lowest LDL level in untreated FH patient was 170 mg/dl (4.4 mmol/l) [9]. Still, there is no question that the higher the LDL-C, the more aggressive the vascular disease.

The second thing is that patients should have a family history of premature atherosclerotic cardiovascular disease (ASCVD), very high cholesterol, or both. Premature ASCVD in a patient is often a clue to FH. In fact, 20% of all myocardial infarctions (MI) in people under the age of 45 are a consequence of FH [17, 18].

The third thing is that the expected response to lipid-lowering therapy is often blunted in FH patients, and their LDL levels are falling less robustly than would normally be anticipated. This occurs because standard medications such as statins and ezetimibe are concentrated on LDLR upregulation. As these receptors by definition defective, their upregulation is less effective at internalizing LDL from plasma.

Physical signs of FH depend greatly on type of the mutation, age, gender, and other factors.

This is an example of one of our FH patient, a 26-year-old woman, who had tendon xanthomas at the age of 1. She have been examined in different clinics (mainly, dermatological), but the diagnosis of FH was suspected only at the age of 10 when concentration of total cholesterol was measured (total cholesterol level = 21 mmol/l) (**Figure 1**).

Unfortunately, LLT (statins, ezetimibe, and LDL-apheresis) has been started in this patient only at the age of 19. She represents positive stress-echo test, and coronary angiography reveals 50% stenosis of the right coronary artery. A 50% stenosis of both common carotid arteries according to an ultrasound was also revealed. At present time, this patient receives 80 mg of atorvastatin, 10 mg of ezetimibe, and LDL-apheresis procedures (each 2 weeks). She also takes part in a randomized placebo-controlled international clinical study on a new *PCSK9* inhibitor—Inclisiran.

You can see a pedigree of this patient in **Figure 2**. It is seen that the index patient (marked with red arrow) with very high cholesterol level has two still young

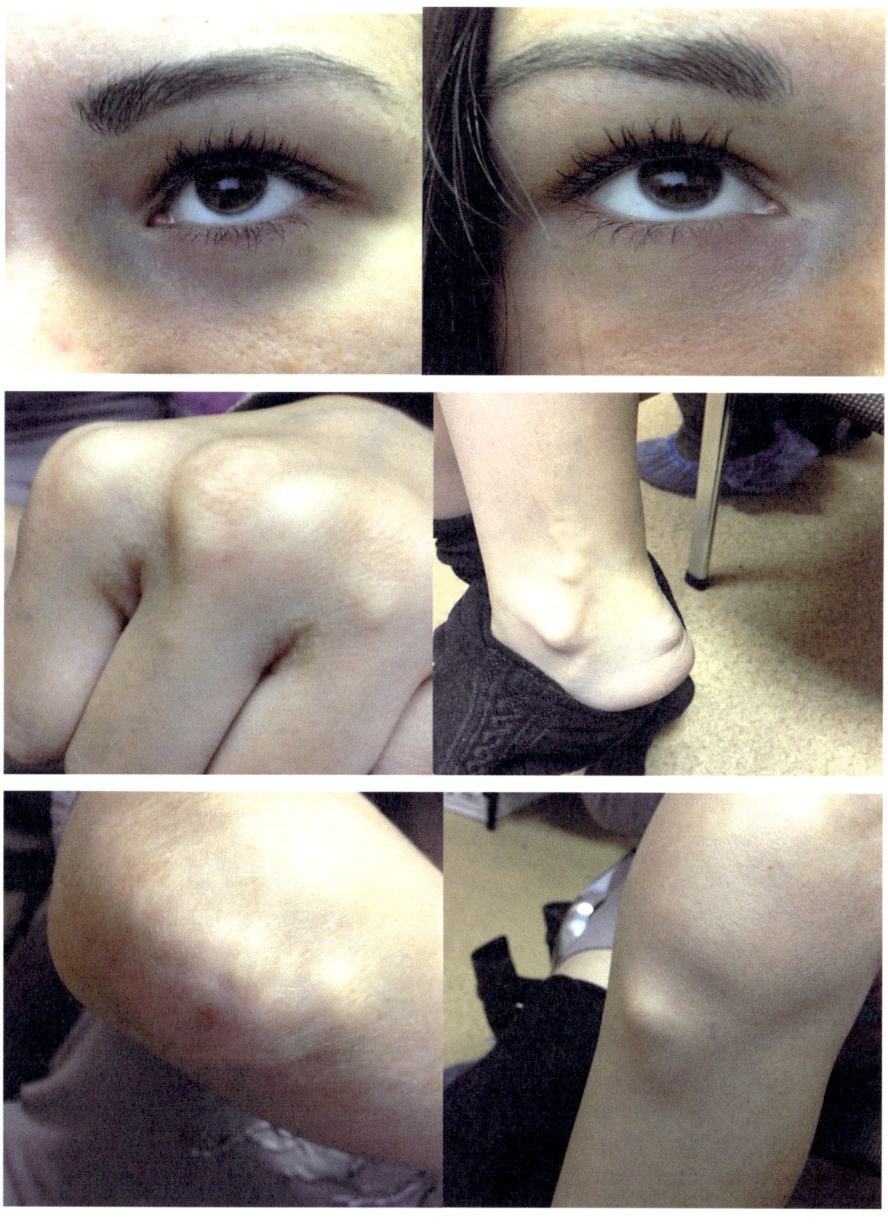

Figure 1.
Corneal arcus (both the eyes) and tendon xanthomas (hands, Achilles tendon, elbow, and knee) in a 26-year-old woman with FH.

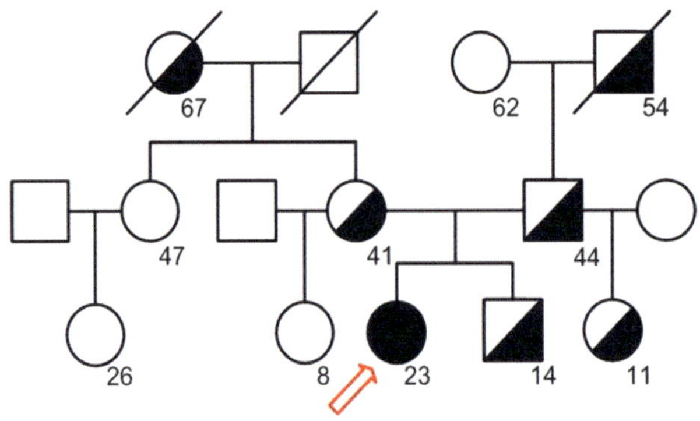

Figure 2.
Pedigree of a 26-year-old female (23 at entry).

parents without clinical signs of ASCVD, but having high total cholesterol levels (9.5–12.2 mmol/l). Parents of proband are divorced, and both of them have new families. The father's daughter from the second marriage who is 11 years of age has also high cholesterol level (8.5 mmol/l). It is seen that the grandfather of the proband died at the age of 54 of acute myocardial infarction (MI).

This patient has undoubtedly homozygous FH phenotype due to a very high cholesterol level, premature atherosclerosis, tendon xanthomas, family history of hypercholesterolemia, and premature ASCVD. Nevertheless, it was interesting to perform genetic testing in this family.

This test was performed in Health-In-Code genetic laboratory (Spain) using Next Generation Sequencing (NGS). Patient specimen (blood) was subjected to automated genomic DNA purification (QIAsymphony SP®, Qiagen). Library preparation was carried out using the Agilent SureSelect library preparation kit for Illumina paired-end multiplexed sequencing according to the manufacturer's instructions. Enrichment of regions of interest was performed using a SureSelect probe kit (Agilent) that selectively captures the coding regions and adjacent intronic areas of the selected genes. After cluster generation, captured DNA was sequenced on the Illumina HiSeq 1500 platform. Sequencing data analysis was done using a proprietary bioinformatics pipeline that includes sample demultiplexing as well as all the steps necessary to obtain a report of annotated variants together with their coverage and corresponding quality parameters.

The design of the custom capture library includes the following six genes related to familial hypercholesterolemia: *APOB, APOE, LDLR, LDLRAP1, PCSK9*, and *SLCO1B1*.

The genes included in this test have been selected on a clinical basis according to their relation to a particular phenotype and classified on the basis of evidence supporting this association into priority, secondary, and candidate genes.

Probes were designed to adequately cover all coding exons and 10 base pairs (bp) of flanking intronic sequences; therefore, this test is unable to identify genetic variants located in intronic zones far from splice sites or UTR regions.

Analysis of SNVs and INDELs: This test can identify single-nucleotide variants (SNVs) and insertions/deletions (INDELs) of up to 20 bp. Genetic variants are reported following the Human Genome Variation Society (HGVS) recommendations (www.hgvs.org).

Genetic variants that are selected because of their potential association with the patient's phenotype or constitute relevant incidental findings are reported in the main table of the report on the first page. Please note that a variant's pathogenicity may be subject to change as new scientific evidence appears.

Confirmation studies: Variants included in the main table meeting the conditions below are confirmed by orthogonal testing:

- point variants (SNVs) and insertions, deletions, and/or INDELs of ≤4 bp that meet at least one of the following criteria: called by only one variant caller, suboptimal quality (QUAL <100), depth of coverage <30x, variants in low-mappability, or multiple alignment regions and
- insertions, deletions, and/or INDELs of >4 bp.

Similarly, low-coverage regions in priority genes that may be of clinical interest are resequenced by the Sanger method.

Analysis of CNVs: Health-In-Code has developed an alternative bioinformatics pipeline that is also able to identify gross insertions/deletions affecting one or more exons of a gene/s included in the panel (CNVs: copy number variations). This complementary analysis is possible when bioinformatics data are adequate (evaluable CNVs) and may not be available in all studies (nonevaluable CNVs).

CNV confirmation studies: Variants identified using this technique will be confirmed by an adequate alternative method.

Analytical specifications of the test: Both analytical sensitivity and specificity of this test are greater than 99% for single-nucleotide variants (SNVs) and insertions/deletions (INDELs) of ≤20 bp.

Average coverage values of the tested gene/s and other quality parameters specific to this patient's study are detailed in each study report.

Technical limitations that can be in any study report: Despite the high sensitivity and specificity of this test, some genotyping errors may occur in specific situations:

- contamination of samples before they arrive at our laboratory;
- mosaic variants;
- monosomies and trisomies;
- genetic paternity problems;
- genetic variants producing allelic drop-outs;
- studies performed on paraffin-embedded tissues;
- presence of pseudogenes (homologous regions);
- incorrect identification of variants in homopolymer or high GC-content zones; and
- errors in the reference sequence

This study is usually not able to identify the phase (same/different alleles) of more than one variant affecting the same gene. This limitation should be considered in cases of recessive disorders, which occur only when both alleles are mutated.

Unequivocal traceability: Health-In-Code developed in-house software NextLIMS that efficiently identifies and tracks samples in the laboratory and allows to unequivocally trace the steps a sample has already gone through.

As you can see in **Figure 3**, two different mutations in the LDLR gene were revealed. First mutation (Val806Glyfs*11) has been previously described and was also found in the mother of proband. Second mutation (Asp569Val) was a new one

RESULT: POSITIVE

Two genetic variants associated or very likely associated with familial hypercholesterolemia have been identified in the LDLR gene. Therefore, in the case that each variant affects a different copy of the gene (a condition called compound heterozygosis), the expected phenotype is clinical homozygous familial hypercholesterolemia (HoHF). We suggest including both of them in the familiar screening to identify other likely to be affected family members. The identification of either variant can be used as a diagnostic criterion for FH in the case that Dutch Lipid Clinic Network or Simon Broome diagnostic criteria are used for evaluation.

Gene	Variant	Result	Pathogenicity	Population frequency	Number of references
LDLR	NP_000518.1:p.Val806Glyfs*11 NM_000527.4:c.2416_2417insG NC_000019.9:g.11240215_11240216insG	Heterozygosis	Pathogenic or disease-causing (+++)	Rare variant (found in <1% of controls)	20
	NP_000518.1:p.Asp569Val NM_000527.4:c.1706A>T NC_000019.9:g.11227535A>T	Heterozygosis	Very likely to be pathogenic or disease-causing (++)	Variant of unknown frequency	0

Other genetic variants possibly not related to the disease have been identified *(see Appendix: Other identified variants).*

Clinical interpretation

The mutation Val806Glyfs*11 has been previously described in association with FH. This mutation affects the protein synthesis and is also called "null allele," or class 1 mutation. This kind of variants are associated with a more severe phenotype and with a poorer response to lipid-lowering drugs compared with other kind of mutations. The mutation Asp569Val has not been previously published, but neither has it been reported in individuals of the general population. It affects a very important region of the LDLR gene where a number of mutations have been clearly associated with FH.

Technical aspects of the study

This sample has been studied by a massive parallel sequencing method using a library that included 6 genes related to familial hypercholesterolemia. Both sensitivity and specificity are above 99% for SNVs and small INDELs (≤20 bp).

Figure 3.
Results of genetic testing in a 26-year-old female, performed in Health-In-Code genetic laboratory (Spain).

(never described in the literature previously). The same mutation was found in a father's daughter from the second marriage. Therefore, in case that each variant affects a different copy of the gene (we call this condition as compound heterozygote), the expected phenotype is homozygous familial hypercholesterolemia.

This clinical case shows difficulties in the diagnosis of FH despite of the presence of obvious facts that actually led to the late onset of LLT and marked atherosclerotic lesions of coronary and carotid arteries in a young patient.

Another patient is a female, 42 years of age with high total cholesterol level (11–12 mmol/l) known for 10 years with no signs of ASCVD. Stress test is negative, intima-media thickness of carotid arteries is 0.8 mm, and no tendon xanthomas or corneal arcus.

It is seen that the father of the proband died at the age of 56 of MI, her aunt at the age of 69 has high cholesterol and angina pectoris, and her cousin at the age of 45 has high cholesterol and underwent CABG (**Figures 4** and **5**).

This clinical case is an example of mutation of *apoB* gene that also leads to hypercholesterolemia. Familial ligand defective apolipoprotein B (FDB) was first described in 1986 by Vega and Grundy [19]. In lipoprotein kinetic studies, it was observed that LDL from some donors was cleared more slowly from circulation in individuals with normal LDL receptor function. Genomic DNA analysis revealed a point mutation in Apo B: CGG-to-CAG mutation at the codon for amino acid 3500 resulting in an arginine to glutamine substitution. The prevalence of this disorder is unknown but is estimated to be 5–10% that seen in FH. Hypercholesterolemia in FDB is usually less severe than in FH. Patients with FDB do respond to statin drug therapy, probably reflecting increased removal of Apo E-containing remnant particles through upregulated hepatic LDL receptors. Our patient was treated with rosuvastatin 40 mg/day + ezetimibe 10 mg/day. Her total cholesterol is 4.9 mmol/l; LDL cholesterol is 2.3 mmol/l; HDL cholesterol is 1.8 mmol/l; and TG is 1.6 mmol/l.

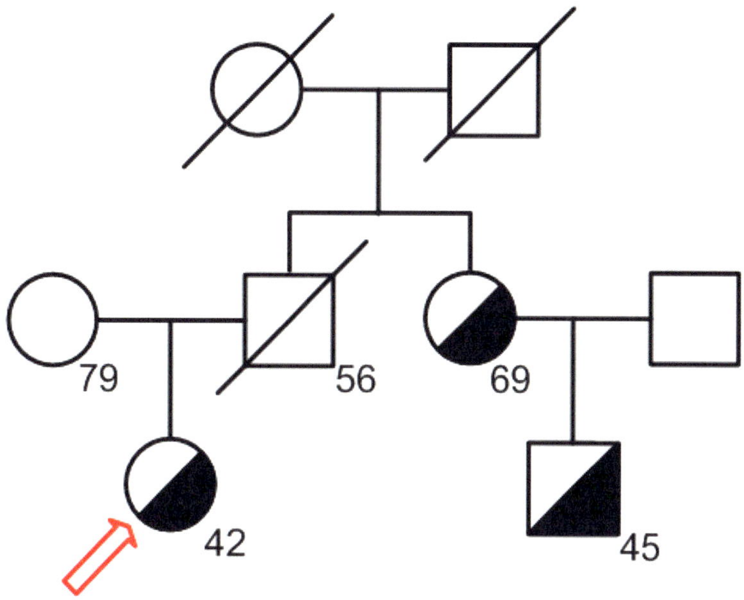

Figure 4.
Pedigree of a 42-year-old woman with high cholesterol level.

RESULT: POSITIVE

We identified a variant in the APOB gene that can explain the patient's phenotype.

Gene	Variant	Result	Pathogenicity	Population frequency	Number of references
APOB	**NP_000375.2:p.Arg3527Gln** **NM_000384.2:c.10580G>A** **NC_000002.11:g.21229160C>T**	Heterozygosis	**Pathogenic or disease-causing (+++)**	**Rare variant (found in <1% of controls)**	205

Other genetic variants possibly not related to the disease have been identified *(see Appendix: Other identified variants).*

Clinical interpretation

The variant identified in the APOB gene is one of the most frequent pathogenic variants known in this gene, which are the cause of familial hypercholesterolemia. The risk of cardiovascular complications is increased. The inclusion of this variant in the familial screening is recommended to evaluate individuals at risk.

This patient also carries the APOE haplotype E4/E3, which may influence the patient's lipid levels or response to lipid-lowering drugs.

Figure 5.
Results of genetic testing in a 42-year-old woman with high cholesterol level.

Physical signs of FH can occur but not needed for the diagnosis. Extensor tendon xanthomas, typically affecting the Achilles or the hands, could appear at the age of 20 and may be present in 70% of older patients. Because xanthomas are subtle, careful examination of the dorsal hand tendons and Achilles tendon is required for their detection. Thus, it is important to always examine the Achilles tendon when performing physical exam. Xanthelasma (cutaneous xanthomas on the palpebra) is common in patients with FH after the age of 30; however, it is not specific for FH. With regard to corneal arcus, it does not have to be circumferential. In fact, it often starts in the superior and inferior aspects of the cornea where the blood supply is greatest. Also, a corneal arcus in someone under 45 years of age is pathognomic for FH [20]. It is important to recognize that because of the prevalent use of lipid-lowering therapy xanthomas, and other clinical signs of FH are uncommon findings nowadays.

Although most FH specialists diagnose FH on clinical grounds, three systems are also available: Make Early Diagnosis to Prevent Early Death (MEDPED), the Dutch Lipid Clinic Network (DLCN), and Simon Broom. Each has its own pros and cons, and none is essential to make the diagnosis. Nevertheless, it is useful to utilize them in clinical practice.

As it is clear from **Table 1**, if a patient has LDL-C level ≥8.5 mmol/l and premature coronary artery or cerebral artery disease, he/she already has more than eight points that means definite FH. It is important to know that if a person has positive results of genetic testing, he/she has only eight points and it is not enough to make a diagnose of definite FH.

Once the diagnosis of FH has been made, he/she is dubbed the proband or the index case. As FH is an autosomal dominant disorder, and early diagnosis and treatment dramatically reduce the risk of future ASCVD events, it is important for physicians to identify other members of the family. Screening relatives of the proband is called "cascade screening."

There are two methods of cascade screening, active and passive. Passive screening employs the index case as the messenger to inform the other family members and recommend further testing. Passive screening is usually not very successful. In contradistinction, active cascade screening—a system in which clinicians rather than patients seek out affected family members—is extraordinarily effective.

	Points
Criteria **Family history**	
First-degree relative with known premature* coronary and vascular disease, OR First-degree relative with known LDL-C level above the 95th percentile	1
First-degree relative with tendinous xanthomata and/or arcus cornealis, OR Children aged less than 18 years with LDL-C level above the 95th percentile	2
Clinical history	
Patient with premature* coronary artery disease	2
Patient with premature* cerebral or peripheral vascular disease	1
Physical examination	
Tendinous xanthomata	6
Arcus cornealis prior to age 45 years	4
Cholesterol levels mg/dl (mmol/liter)	
LDL-C >= 330 mg/dL (≥8.5)	8
LDL-C 250 – 329 mg/dL (6.5–8.4)	5
LDL-C 190 – 249 mg/dL (5.0–6.4)	3
LDL-C 155 – 189 mg/dL (4.0–4.9)	1
DNA analysis	
Functional mutation in the *LDLR, apo B or PCSK9* gene	8
Diagnosis (diagnosis is based on the total number of points obtained)	
Definite Familial Hypercholesterolemia	>8
Probable Familial Hypercholesterolemia	6 – 8
Possible Familial Hypercholesterolemia	3 – 5
Unlikely Familial Hypercholesterolemia	<3

**Premature = <55 years in men; <60 years in women.*
LDL-C, low-density lipoprotein cholesterol; LDLR, low-density lipoprotein receptor; apoB, *apolipoprotein B;* PCSK9, *proprotein convertase subtilisin/kexin type 9.*

Table 1.
Dutch Lipid Clinic Network Score for FH [21–23].

It was successfully performed in the Netherlands. This active cascade screening system sets the bar for the world, identifying nearly 75% of the Netherland's FH population and adding eight additional FH patients for every single-index case identified [9].

The time course of FH depends on a lot of genetic and environmental factors. Previously, we have identified mutations of the LDLR gene in 45 families in St. Petersburg [24]. Our aim was to follow the development of dyslipidemia in children of probands with verified mutations of the LDLR gene as these children were growing up, to compare severity of atherosclerotic complications in patients with different LDLR gene mutations, and to compare atherosclerotic disease progress in males and females with FH. We were following probands with FH and their available relatives with LDLR gene mutations, including children, during 10 years. In all patients, total blood plasma cholesterol, triglycerides, LDL cholesterol, and HDL cholesterol were monitored, and clinical manifestations of ASCVD were documented.

As it is seen in **Table 2**, there were 26 original mutations of the LDLR gene, and 7 were not original but revealed in different families. Due to high heterogeneity of FH-causing mutation in St. Petersburg, we failed to establish interrelations between type of LDLR gene mutation and severity of atherosclerosis manifestation. As a rule, complications of coronary artery disease (CAD) were found less commonly and tend to be less severe in females rather than in males (**Table 3**).

As you can see in **Table 3**, CAD was revealed in three-fourth of males with LDLR gene mutations and only in half of females. Thus, mean age of healthy persons was 34 ± 3.1 years in males and 41 ± 2.6 years in females. Mean age of patients with CAD clinical manifestations was 45 ± 1.9 and 53 ± 2.9, respectively. Otherwise, males suffer from atherosclerotic complications more frequently and much earlier than females. Apparently, females are defended of ASCVD anyway in cases of FH. Some authors explain this by protective function of estrogens. Not infrequently, this protection still remains in the menopause period. To our mind, this protective effect could be explained by the level of HDL cholesterol. Thus, we followed up a mother and her two daughters with genetically verified diagnosis of FH. Mother and her younger daughter had severe clinical manifestations of CAD, while older daughter had no clinical manifestations of ASCVD and did not take LLT. LDL levels did not differ

Number of probands with LDLR gene mutations	Number of members of families of probands with LDLR gene mutations	Number of original mutations (revealed only in one family)	Number of families with the same type of LDLR gene mutation in two families	Number of families with the same (only one) mutation (G197del)
45	78	26	6 (12 probands, 6 variants of the LDLR gene mutation)	7 probands with 1 variant of mutation

Table 2.
Number of probands and their relatives with LDLR gene mutations.

Gender	Number of patients	Patients with CAD	Mean age of patients with CAD	Patients without CAD	Mean age of patients without CAD
Male	26	20	45 ± 1.9	6	34 ± 3.1
Female	38	19	53 ± 2.9	19	41 ± 2.6

Table 3.
Number of males and females with the LDLR gene mutations, their age, and the presence of coronary heart disease.

Groups of patients (see text)	Number of patients	LDL/HDL
Group 1	15	10.4 ± 0.78
Group 2	8	7.7 ± 0.89
Group 3	10	5.2 ± 0.45

Difference between Groups 1 and 2 and Groups 2 and 3 is statistically significant ($p<0.05$).

Table 4.
LDL/HDL ratio in the three groups of patients with LDLR gene mutations.

greatly in the members of this family (326 mg/dl—mother, 322 mg/dl—younger daughter (24-year-old), 277 mg/dl—older daughter (30-year-old)), while HDL-C was 44 mg/dl and 49 mg/dl in the first two woman and 65 mg/dl—in the third.

We divided patients with LDLR gene mutations into three groups (**Table 4**). 1 with progressive CAD, 2 with stable disease, 3 without clinical manifestation of CAD and measured LDL/HDL ratio.

It is seen that high level of HDL is the only one proved lipid factor preventing atherosclerosis development in patients with genetically verified familial hypercholesterolemia.

3. Conclusion

Management of FH must always begin with therapeutic lifestyle changes (TLC); therefore, TLC is the foundation of all ASCVD prevention [25]. A healthful diet limited in saturated fats and simple sugars, daily aerobic exercise, avoidance of tobacco and alcohol, maintenance of an optimal blood pressure and weight, and reduction of stress are all important. The mainstay of therapy in FH is to lower the LDL-C as much and as soon as possible. One must remember that all patients with FH are considered high cardiovascular risk, and for this reason, formal risk stratification with Framingham or Score systems is never advised when guiding treatment. According to the European Guidelines, the goal of lipid-lowering therapy is <1.4 mmol/l if the patient has CAD, diabetes mellitus or >50% stenosis of carotid or peripheral arteries, and <1.8 mmol/l—without clinical manifestations of ASCVD [26]. It is recommended in adult patients to use high intensive statin therapy (atorvastatin 80 mg or rosuvastatin 40 mg). In cases where the goal is not achieved on statin therapy, it is recommended to add ezetimibe 10 mg. If the goal is not achieved, you should think about adding *PCSK9* inhibitors (alirocumab 75/150 mg each 2 weeks, evolocumab 140 mg each 2 weeks or 420 mg once a month).

Drug therapy in children with FH should be started at the age of 8–10 years. The LDL-C goal is <4.0 mmol/l (8–10 years) and <3.5 mmol/l (10 years and more). Treatment should be started with statins. In case of homozygous FH when LDL-C levels are more than 13 mmol/l and ASCVD appears in childhood, the treatment should be started from a maximal doses of statins with the addition of ezetimibe and evolocumab (in children >12 years). In severe cases of HoFH, extracorporeal methods of treatment (LDL apheresis, HELP, etc.) are recommended.

Despite of the fact that pathogenesis and clinical manifestations of FH are well understood, this disease still remains underdiagnosed and undertreated. All FH patients are to be considered high risk. Some, however, are unfortunately even higher risk than rest. It depends on age, gender, or some biochemical and environmental risk and antirisk factors. Early diagnosis and management of FH can significantly improve lifespan and quality of life in these patients.

Author details

Vladimir O. Konstantinov
Department of Internal Medicine and Cardiology, Metchnikov North-West State Medical University, Saint-Petersburg, Russian Federation

*Address all correspondence to: atherosclerosis@mail.ru

References

[1] Goldstein JL, Hobbs HH, Brown MS. Familial hypercholesterolemia. In: Scriver CR, Beaudet AL, Sly WS, et al., editors. The Metabolic and Molecular Bases of Inherited Disease. 8th ed. New York: McGraw-Hill; 2001. pp. 2863-2913

[2] Bredie SJ, Kiemeney LA, de Haan AF, et al. Inherited susceptibility determines the distribution of dense low-density lipoprotein subfraction profiles in familial combined hyperlipidemia. American Journal of Human Genetics. 1996;**58**:812-822

[3] Goldstein JL, Brown MS. Familial hypercholesterolemia: Identification of a defect in the regulation of 3-hydroxy-3methylglutaril coenzyme A reductase activity associated with overproduction of cholesterol. Proceedings of the National Academy of Sciences of the United States of America. 1973;**70**(10):2804-2808

[4] Brown MS, Goldstein GL. Familial hypercholesterolemia: Defective binding of lipoproteins to cultured fibroblasts associated with impaired regulation of 3-hydroxy-3-methylglutaril coenzyme A reductase activity. Proceedings of the National Academy of Sciences of the United States of America. 1974;**71**(3):788-792

[5] Cuchel M et al. Homozygous familial hypercholesterolemia: New insights and guidance for clinicians to improve detection and clinical management. A position paper from the Consensus Panel on Familial Hypercholesterolemia of the European Atherosclerosis Society. European Heart Journal. 2014;**35**(32):2146-2157

[6] Boren J et al. The molecular mechanism for the genetic disorder familial defective apolipoprotein B100. The Journal of Biological Chemistry. 2001;**276**(12):9214-9218

[7] Whitfield AJ et al. Lipid disorders and mutations in the APOB gene. Clinical Chemistry. 2004;**50**(10):1725-1732

[8] Horton JD, Cohen JC, Hobbs HH. Molecular biology of PCSK9: Its role in LDL metabolism. Trends in Biochemical Sciences. 2007;**32**(2):71-77

[9] Sjouke B et al. Homozygous autosomal dominant hypercholesterolemia in the Netherlands: Prevalence, genotype-phenotype relationship, and clinical outcome. European Heart Journal. 2015;**36**(9):560-565

[10] Vishwanath R, Hemphill LC. Familial hypercholesterolemia and estimation of US patients eligible for low-density lipoprotein apheresis after maximally tolerated lipid-lowering therapy. Journal of Clinical Lipidology. 2014;**8**(1):18-28

[11] Walzer S et al. Homozygous familial hypercholesterolemia (HoFH) in Germany: An epidemiological survey. Clinicoecon Outcomes Research. 2013;**5**:189-192

[12] Seftel HC et al. Prevalence of familial hypercholesterolemia in Johannesburg Jews. American Journal of Medical Genetics. 1989;**34**(4):545-547

[13] Zakharova FM, Damgaard D, Mandelshtam MY, Golubkov VI, et al. Familial hypercholesterolemia in St-Petersburg: The known and novel mutations found in the low-density lipoprotein receptor gene in Russia. BMC Medical Genetics. 2005;**8**:6-6

[14] Marais AD et al. A dose-titration and comparative study of rosuvastatin and atorvastatin in patients with homozygous familial hypercholesterolemia. Atherosclerosis. 2008;**197**(1):400-406

[15] Raal FJ, Santos RD. Homozygous familial hypercholesterolemia:

Current perspectives on diagnosis and treatment. Atherosclerosis. 2012;**223**(2):262-268

[16] Kolansky DM et al. Longitudinal evaluation and assessment of cardiovascular disease in patients with homozygous familial hypercholesterolemia. The American Journal of Cardiology. 2008;**102**(11):1438-1443

[17] Goldstein JL et al. Hyperlipidemia and coronary heart disease. II. Genetic analysis of lipid levels in 176 families and delineation of a new inherited disorder, combined hyperlipidemia. The Journal of Clinical Investigation. 1973;**52**(7):1544-1568

[18] Neefjes LA et al. Accelerated subclinical coronary atherosclerosis in patients with familial hypercholesterolemia. Atherosclerosis. 2011;**219**(2):721-727

[19] Vega GL, Grundy SM. In vivo evidence for reduced binding of low density lipoproteins to receptors as a cause of primary moderate hypercholesterolemia. The Journal of Clinical Investigation. 1986;**78**:1410-1414

[20] Zech LA, Hoeg GM. Correlating corneal arcus with atherosclerosis in familial hypercholesterolemia. Lipids in Health and Disease. 2008;7:7

[21] Austin MA, Hutter CM, Zimmern RL, Humphries SE. Genetic causes of monogenic heterozygous familial hypercholesterolemia: A HuGE prevalence review. American Journal of Epidemiology. 2004;**160**:407-420

[22] Haase A, Goldberg AC. Identification of people with heterozygous familial hypercholesterolemia. Current Opinion in Lipidology. 2012;**23**:282-289

[23] Nordestgaard BG, Chapman MJ, Humphries SE, et al. Familial hypercholesterolemia is underdiagnosed and undertreated in the general population: Guidance for clinicians to prevent coronary heart disease: Consensus statement of the European Atherosclerosis Society. European Heart Journal. 2013;**34**:3478-3490a

[24] Lipovetsky BM, Mandelshtam MY, Konstantinov VO. Clinico-genetical peculiarities of probands with familial hypercholesterolemia and members of their families, observed during 10 years and more. Atherosclerosis and Dyslipidemias. 2015;**1**:41-46. Russian

[25] Eckel RH et al. AHA/ACC guideline on lifestyle management to reduce cardiovascular risk: A report of the American College of Cardiology/ American Heart Association Task Force on Practice Guidelines. Journal of the American College of Cardiology. 2013, 2014;**63**(25PtB):2960-2984

[26] Mach F, Baigent C, Catapano AL, et al. ESC/EAS Guidelines for the management of dyslipidemias: Lipid modification to reduce cardiovascular risk. European Heart Journal. 2020;**41**(1):111-188

Section 3

A Therapeutic Approach to Vascular Pathologies

Chapter 5

Statin Therapy in Children

Bhuvana Sunil and Ambika Pallikunnath Ashraf

Abstract

Landmark studies such as the Bogalusa Heart study, Pathobiological Determinants of Atherosclerosis in Youth study, and Muscatine and Young Finns studies established that the atherosclerotic process begins in childhood. Early precursors of atherosclerosis may increase risk of cardiovascular morbidity in adulthood. Follow-up studies of children with familial homozygous hypercholesterolemia showed that initiation of statin therapy slowed the progression of carotid intima-media thickness and reduced cardiovascular disease risk. Despite the growing evidence on the efficacy of statins and a rising prevalence of dyslipidemia, there are concerns regarding long-term safety and efficacy. Moreover, data on statin use in children with secondary dyslipidemia are sparse. This chapter provides a comprehensive review of the current state of literature on the indications, contraindications, efficacy and safety data on the use of statins in pediatric dyslipidemia.

Keywords: pediatric dyslipidemia, HMG Co-A reductase inhibitors, low-density lipoprotein cholesterol, cardiovascular risk factors

1. Introduction

Cardiovascular disease (CVD) is the leading cause of mortality in the United States [1]. Atherosclerosis, a silent precursor of CVD has its origins from early in childhood [2, 3]. Some dyslipidemias such as familial hypercholesterolemia (FH) and familial combined hyperlipidemia (FCH) are highly prevalent clinically silent disorders. Elevated lipid levels in childhood track well into adulthood [4]. In 2011, the National Heart, Lung, and Blood Institute (NHLBI) convened an expert panel on Cardiovascular Health and Risk Reduction in Children and Adolescents, which recommended for universal lipid screening in the pediatric population [5]. The universal lipid screening leads to identification of a large number of children with previously unrecognized dyslipidemia. Statins are one of the most potent classes of lipid lowering medications for CV risk reduction. This chapter describes the current screening and management guidelines, efficacy and adverse effects of statin therapy in pediatric dyslipidemia.

1.1 Mechanism of action of statins

The primary mechanism of action of statins is inhibition of the enzyme-3-hydroxy-3-methylglutaryl-coenzyme A (HMG-CoA) reductase. This is a rate-limiting step in the biosynthesis of cholesterol. Reduced intrahepatic cholesterol leads to decreased VLDL assembly. The hepatocyte cholesterol depletion leads to upregulation of sterol regulatory binding element proteins (SREBPs), the nuclear transcription factors that regulate LDL receptors (LDL-R). Upregulation of LDL-R on the surface of the hepatocyte in turn results in increased uptake and degradation of low-density lipoprotein cholesterol (LDL) [6]. They reduce the secretion of apoB, which affects the rate at which HMG CoA reductase is available to synthesize cholesterol again [7].

Statins induce inhibition of the Rho-signaling pathway, activate peroxisome proliferator-activated receptor alpha (PPARα) and improve HDL levels by increased production of apoA-I, the major apolipoprotein of HDL [8, 9]. Decrease in isoprenylation of signaling molecules, such as Ras, Rho, and Rac, leads to the modulation of various signaling pathways. By inhibiting mevalonic acid synthesis, statins prevent the synthesis of isoprenoid intermediates farnesyl pyrophosphate and geranyl geranylpyrophosphate [10]. It has been long established that a pro-inflammatory environment is necessary for plaque progression and advancement of atherosclerosis, and these intermediates are known to have a pro-inflammatory effect. Statins can inhibit posttranslational modification of Ras and Rho, which regulate cell proliferation, differentiation, apoptosis, and the cytoskeletal modifications [11]. Statins have also been proposed to be beneficial to prevent progression of atherosclerosis by their pleiotropic effect [12]. Experimental models have suggested reduction in T-cell clustering with the use of statins, thereby proposing an immunomodulatory effect [13].

1.2 Risk factors and medical conditions

Table 1 lists the medical risk factors and conditions to be considered while screening for dyslipidemia as defined by the Expert Panel on Integrated Guidelines for Cardiovascular Health and Risk Reduction in Children and Adolescents. The terminology from this table will be used throughout the chapter.

1.3 Current screening recommendations for pediatric dyslipidemia

Although the atherosclerotic process begins in childhood, most pediatric lipid disorders do not have any obvious clinical manifestations [2, 3]. Screening based on family history alone can miss up to 30–60% dyslipidemias [5, 14]. In higher risk

Positive family history: parent, grandparent, aunt, uncle, sibling with any of these before the age 55 Y in a male or 65 Y in a female: myocardial infarction, stroke, angina, coronary artery bypass, stent, angioplasty, sudden cardiac death, parent with total cholesterol >240 mg/dL	
High risk factors: • Hypertension requiring drug therapy (BP ≥ 99th%ile + 5 mmHg) • Current cigarette smoker • BMI ≥ 97th%ile	**Moderate risk factors**: • Hypertension not requiring drug therapy • BMI ≥ 95th%ile, < 97th%ile • HDL–C < 40 mg/dL
High risk medical conditions: • Diabetes mellitus, type 1 and type 2 • Chronic renal disease/end-stage renal disease/postrenal transplant • Postorthotopic heart transplant • Kawasaki disease with current aneurysms	**Moderate risk medical conditions**: • Kawasaki disease with regressed coronary aneurysms • Chronic inflammatory disease • Human immunodeficiency virus (HIV) infection • Nephrotic syndrome

Abbreviations: BP, blood pressure; BMI, body mass index.
Adapted from Expert Panel on Integrated Guidelines for Cardiovascular Health and Risk Reduction in Children and Adolescents, National Heart, Lung, and Blood Institute 2011.

Table 1.
Cardiovascular risk factors and high-risk medical conditions.

adult patients, especially those with disorders such as FH, statin therapy has been retrospectively associated with reducing risk of major cardiovascular events [15]. In the absence of clear history or physical examination findings, recognition of children with lipid disorders needs universal screening. The United States NHLBI, the American Academy of Pediatrics and the American Heart Association have all endorsed selective risk based screening and universal screening [5, 16, 17]. International Organizations such as the European Atherosclerosis Society recommend selective and cascade screening [18]. In contrast, the United States Preventive Services Task Force (USPSTF) concluded that current evidence is insufficient to assess the benefits or harms of screening for lipid disorders in children and adolescents, even though it acknowledges the importance of early identification of dyslipidemias [19]. For many CV risk factors like dyslipidemia, hypertension, and obesity, it is difficult to conduct large, long-term studies because of the time, cost and expected difficulties in study adherence. Recently, relatively long term follow up studies indicated that the initiation of statin therapy during childhood in patients with FH slowed the progression of carotid intima-media thickness and reduced the risk of cardiovascular disease in adulthood [20].

Screening can be performed either with a fasting or non-fasting serum lipid profile. The triglyceride (TG) levels are the most affected component of the lipid profile by non-fasting status. The LDL and non-HDL (TC-HDL) are mostly unaffected by the non-fasting status and can therefore be used for screening purposes [21, 22]. Cholesterol and LDL tend to increase until 2 years and plateau until adolescence. A 10–20% reduction of TC and LDL occurs in both normal children as well as children with genetic dyslipidemias during puberty, and can result in false negatives during this time [23]. Therefore, it is important to universally screen for lipid disorders between ages 9–11 Y and repeat between ages 17–19 Y. **Table 2** depicts lipid values very by age, according National Cholesterol Education Program (NCEP) Expert Panel on Cholesterol Levels in Children.

Up to 12 months, no routine screening of lipid profiles is recommended in infancy. Between 2 and 8 Y and 12 and 16 Y, a fasting lipid profile (FLP) is recommended if there is a positive family history, if the child has a moderate or high-risk medical condition or a high risk factor. Between 9 and 11 Y and 17 and 21 Y, universal screening is recommended. If on a non-fasting sample, the non-HDL $\geq$ 145 mg/dL or HDL < 40 mg/dL, it is recommended to repeat an FLP twice within 2 weeks to 3 months and average the results. Values to address on the FLP

Categories	Acceptable	Borderline high	High
Total cholesterol	<170	171–199	>200
LDL	<110	110–129	≥130
Non-HDL	<120	120–144	≥145
TG (0–9 Y)	<75	75–99	≥100
TG (10–19 Y)	<90	90–129	≥130
HDL	>45	40–45	<40

Abbreviations: TC, total cholesterol; LDL, low-density lipoprotein cholesterol; HDL, high-density lipoprotein cholesterol; TG, triglyceride.
Values from the National Cholesterol Education Program [24]. All fasting values in mg/dL. To convert to SI units, divide total cholesterol, LDL, HDL, and non-HDL by 38.6, and for TG, divide by 88.6.
High and borderline-high values are indicative of approximately the 95th and 75th percentiles for age.

Table 2.
Lipid values by age.

after averaging the results include LDL ≥ 130 mg/dL, non-HDL ≥ 145 mg/dL, HDL < 40 mg/dL, TG ≥ 100 mg/dL if <10 years; ≥ 130 mg/dL if ≥10 years [5].

1.4 Diagnostic considerations in pediatric dyslipidemia

Dyslipidemia could be primary or secondary. Primary lipid disorders include monogenic conditions like FH or familial hypertriglyceridemia. Some genetic dyslipidemias like FCH do not have a recognized genetic defect yet, and have variable degrees of dyslipidemia and varying patterns of increase of TG and LDL within the same family. Obesity can exacerbate the expression of dyslipidemia in children with this underlying genotype. Lipid disorders could also be secondary to the underlying untreated medical conditions. Some considerations include diabetes mellitus, hypothyroidism, hypercortisolism, metabolic syndrome, growth hormone deficiency, pregnancy, drug and medication use, acute and chronic hepatitis, nephrotic syndrome, chronic kidney disease etc. [25–31].

After ruling out secondary dyslipidemias, primary dyslipidemias are to be considered. Primary lipid disorders can be broadly categorized by the predominantly affected component of the lipid profile. **Table 3** depicts patterns of inheritance, predominant affected lipoprotein and prevalence in the more commonly encountered primary dyslipidemias. Of these conditions, the most prevalent conditions are heterozygous FH (HeFH 1:300) and FCH (1:100).

1.5 Lifestyle management of dyslipidemia

Dietary management and lifestyle changes are the cornerstone of therapy for many secondary dyslipidemias. A registered dietitian nutritionist is central to implementing lifestyle changes, trained to assess the child's nutritional status and make practical modifications to facilitate behavioral changes. In children and adolescents with obesity, moderate, gradual weight reduction has been shown to improve dyslipidemia and decrease insulin resistance.

The NCEP has proposed a stepwise dietary regulation for children with elevated LDL levels. For all children more than 1 year of age and older, the Cardiovascular Health Integrated Lifestyle Diet (CHILD)-1 diet is the first step (Step 1 diet); this constitutes total fat (25–30% of total daily calories), saturated fat (8–10% of daily kcal/estimated energy requirements), avoiding trans-fat, <300 mg/day from cholesterol, dietary fiber (14 g/1000 kcal), fat-free unflavored milk, limiting sodium intake and sweetened juice (no added sugar) <120 mL/day. Polyunsaturated fatty acids up to 10% of daily calories, and monounsaturated fatty acid intake of 10–15% of daily caloric intake is recommended [5].

If the CHILD-1 modifications do not show the desired lipid changes within 3 months of initiation, the next step is to advance to the CHILD-2 diet (Step 2 diet), which further restricts saturated fat. The CHILD-2 diet consists of 25–30% of total calories from fat, <7% from saturated fat, <10% from monounsaturated fat, and avoiding trans-fat. The CHILD-2 diet specific for LDL lowering (CHILD-2-LDL) also recommends use of fiber supplementation and plant stanols/sterols: plant sterol and stanol esters up to 2 g/day, water-soluble fiber psyllium, dose of 6 g/day (2–12 years) and 12 g/day (>12 years). The CHILD 2 diet specific to TG lowering (CHILD-2-TG) recommends decreasing sugar and sugar-sweetened beverages, replacing simple with complex carbohydrates, and increasing dietary fish to increase omega-3 fatty acid intake [5].

The expert panel also recommends at least 1 h of moderate-to vigorous physical activity every day of the week, with vigorous, intense physical activity on at least 3

Name	Genetic defect	Pattern of inheritance	Incidence	Lipid profile/lipoprotein pattern
		Disorders with elevated LDL		
Familial homozygous hypercholesterolemia	LDL-R Gain of function PCSK9 Familial defective apo B-*100*	AD	1:1,000,000	↑↑ ↑ TC ↑ ↑ LDL
Familial heterozygous hypercholesterolemia	Same as above	AR	1:300–400	↑ TC ↑ LDL
Autosomal recessive hypercholesterolemia	LDL-R Adaptor protein	AR	<1:1,000,000	↑ TC ↑ LDL
Sitosterolemia	*ABCG5* *ABCG8*	AR	<1:1,000,000	↑ TC ↑ LDL ↑ serum sitosterol, campesterol
Lysosomal acid lipase deficiency	LIPA gene defect	AR	1:40,000–300,000	↑ LDL
Cholesterol 7α-Hydroxylase deficiency	CYP7A1 gene	Semi-dominant	<1:1,000,000	↑ TC ↑ LDL ↑TG
Familial combined hyperlipidemia	Unknown	AD	1:100–200	↑ TC ↑ LDL ↑VLDL ↑TG, Chylomicrons, ↑ VLDL remnants
Dysbetalipoproteinemia	apoE	AR	1:5000	↑ ↑ TC ↑ ↑ LDL ↑↑ IDL ↑↑ TG ↑ Chylomicrons
		Disorders with elevated TG		
Familial hypertriglyceridemia	Unknown	AD	1:500	↑ TC ↑↑ TG
Familial chylomicronemia	LPL deficiency apoC-II deficiency apoA5 and *GPIHBP1* loss-of-function	AR	1 out of 1,000,000	↑ TC ↑↑↑ TG
		Disorders with reduced HDL		
Hypoalphalipoproteinemia	APOA1	AD	<1:1,000,000	↓ HDL ↓ or normal TG
Tangier disease	ABCA1	AR	<1:1,000,000	↓ HDL normal or ↑ TG
Lecithin cholesterol acyl transferase deficiency	*LCAT* (16q22.1)	AR	<1:1,000,000	↓ HDL

Abbreviations: TC, total cholesterol; LDL, low density lipoprotein cholesterol; HDL, high density lipoprotein cholesterol; TG, triglyceride; AD, autosomal dominant; AR, autosomal recessive; LDL-R, LDL receptor; PCSK9, proprotein convertase subtilisin/kexin type 9; apoB, apolipoprotein; ABCG, ATP-binding cassette sub-family G member; LIPA, lysosomal acid lipase type A; LPL, lipoprotein lipase; GPIHBP1, *glycosylphosphatidylinositol anchored high density lipoprotein binding protein 1;* LCAT, *lecithin cholesterol acyl transferase.*

Table 3.
Characteristic features of primary dyslipidemias.

of these days in agreement with the 2008 Physical Activity Guidelines for Americans from the U.S. [5].

1.6 Laboratory evaluations prior to statin therapy

Suggested serum testing prior to initiation of statin therapy include testing to rule out secondary causes of dyslipidemia—serum albumin, blood glucose level or hemoglobin A1C, renal function tests, serum thyroid-stimulating hormone, free T4 concentration, and a pregnancy screen. These tests are to be done as deemed clinically necessary. Liver function studies, serum creatinine kinase (CK) levels are useful to obtain at baseline to monitor for future potential adverse effects.

1.7 Indications for statin therapy in pediatrics

Children with average LDL-C ≥ 190 mg/dL have a high likelihood of FH and almost certainly require pharmacotherapy, as diet and exercise modifications can maximally reduce lipids by ~10–20% [32]. Fasting TG level of ≥500 mg/dL (which may indicate postprandial elevations to >1000 mg/dL and risk of pancreatitis) are also best referred and managed by a lipid specialist. Referral may ultimately be required if LDL levels remain elevated beyond ≥160 mg/dL despite 6 months of lifestyle interventions. Once the lipid profile has been repeated within a 2 week to 3-month period, the following average values currently are recommended to start statin therapy concomitantly with diet and lifestyle modifications.

In children <10 years of age:

- Homozygous familial hypercholesterolemia (HoFH) with LDL typically above 400 mg/dL
- CVD within the first two decades of life/post cardiac transplantation
- LDL ≥190 mg/dL + positive family history, OR 1 high risk factor/condition, OR 2 moderate risk factors/conditions

In children ≥10 years:

- LDL ≥ 190 mg/dL
- LDL ≥ 160 mg/dL + positive family history, OR 1 high risk factor/condition, OR 2 moderate risk factors/conditions
- LDL ≥130 mg/dL + 2 high risk factors/conditions, OR 1 high risk factor/condition and 2 moderate risk factors/conditions, OR clinical CVD

1.8 Expected effects of statin therapy

Aside from PCSK9 inhibitors, statins are the most potent class of lipid lowering agents. The expected effects of statin therapy on TC and LDL levels are dependent on their potency and dosing. Most statins have a mild effect on increasing HDL by 2–5%, and on decreasing TG levels by up to 40%. **Table 4** outlines the starting dosing, properties and potency by expected effects on LDL reduction of some of the commonly used statins in pediatrics. Although the statins with longer half-lives inhibit the enzyme for a longer time, even with statins that have a shorter half-life are effective at reducing the LDL levels because they reduce overall serum levels of lipoproteins with a half-life of approximately 2–3 days. For this reason, all statins can be administered in once a day dosing. The general principal behind statin therapy in pediatrics is to use the lowest effective doses of a statin. Currently, the maximum daily dose studied in pediatrics is for 40 mg of lovastatin, pravastatin, and simvastatin; 20 mg of atorvastatin and rosuvastatin; and 80 mg of fluvastatin.

Statin	Typical dose (mg)	Maximum dose (mg)	Half-life (h)	Lipophilicity	Fecal excretion (%)	Renal excretion (%)	Effect on LDL reduction (%)
Atorvastatin	5–10	80	15–30	Lipophilic	>98	<2	38–54
Fluvastatin	20	80	0.5–2.3	Lipophilic	93	6	17–33
Lovastatin	10	80	2.9	Lipophilic	83	10	29–48
Pravastatin	5–20	40	1.3–2.8	Hydrophilic	70	20	19–40
Rosuvastatin	5–10	40	19	Hydrophilic	90	10	52–63
Simvastatin	5–10	40	2–3	Lipophilic	60	13	28–41

Abbreviation: LDL, low-density lipoprotein cholesterol.

Table 4.
Starting doses and properties of statin drug therapy.

In the United States, pravastatin and pitavastatin have FDA approval for children age ≥ 8 years with HeFH. Lovastatin, simvastatin, fluvastatin, atorvastatin and rosuvastatin have been approved for children ≥10 years with FH. At the higher prescribed doses, atorvastatin and rosuvastatin are more potent than the other approved medications [33]. Key randomized clinical trials for each of these statins in the order of approval for pediatric use are summarized in **Table 5**.

1.9 Special considerations for high-risk conditions

As diabetes is considered a CV risk factor, intensive lipid management is suggested for these patients. In addition to maintaining the best glycemic control possible, the American Diabetes Association recommends starting treatment with statins for LDL ≥ 160 mg/dL and considering treatment for LDL ≥ 130 mg/dL with additional risk factors basing the treatment decision on the child's complete CVD risk profile, including assessment of blood pressure, family history, and smoking status with a goal of lowering LDL to under 100 mg/dL [48].

In nephrotic syndrome, chronic kidney disease and polycystic ovarian syndrome as well LDL ≥ 160 mg/dL maybe a threshold for initiating statin treatment in addition to adequate mediation therapy for the underlying condition, lifestyle and diet therapy. In Kawasaki disease, patients >2 years old without persistent coronary artery abnormalities should undergo lipid screening 1 year after the acute phase, and if normal, universal screening can be considered. Patients with coronary artery aneurysms should undergo annual screening and treated for levels ≥160 mg/dL.

1.10 Challenges in pediatric dosing

Thus far, statins are only available in pill form. With the exception of simvastatin oral suspension, other liquid preparations or flavoring are not readily available which maybe an issue for children with sensory issues or difficulty swallowing a pill. A disintegrating formulation of simvastatin is available, and this may be helpful in younger children. Although compounding the medication at local pharmacies is an option, several logistical issues limit this accessibility. Some of the extended release preparations such as Lovastatin and fluvastatin are rarely used in children, and should not be crushed. Fluvastatin is available as a capsule but the contents are not to be separated per manufacturer's instructions.

Group	Study design	Test group	N	Age	Condition	Duration	Outcomes
				Atorvastatin			
McCrindle et al. [34]	Placebo controlled RCT	10–20 mg	187	10–17 Y	HeFH or severe hypercholesterolemia	6 months	TC ↓ 32% LDL ↓ 40% TG ↓ 12% ApoB ↓ 34% HDL ↑ 2.8%
Gandelman et al. [35]	No	5–10 mg	39	6–10 Y (TS 1) 10–18 Y (TS 2)	HeFH	8 weeks	TC ↓ 34.1–35.6% LDL ↓ 40.7–39.7% TG ↓ 6–21.1%
Canas et al. [36]	Placebo controlled RCT	10–20 mg	42	10–20Y	T1D	6 months	TC ↓ 21% LDL ↓ 32% Non-HDL ↓ 31% ApoB ↓ 26%
Langslet et al. [37]	No	5 mg or 10 mg, ↑ up to 80 mg	272	6–15 Y	HeFH	3 years	LDL ↓ 43.8% TS 1 and 39.9% for TS ≥2
				Fluvastatin			
Van der Graaf et al. [38]	No—single arm study	80 mg	85	10–16 Y	HeFH	2 years	TC ↓ 27.1% LDL ↓ 33.9% TG ↓ 5.3% ApoB ↓ 24.2%
				Lovastatin			
Lambert et al. [39]	Controlled multicenter RCT	10, 20, 30 and 40 mg doses	69	<17Y (boys only)	FH	8 weeks	TC ↓ 17–29% LDL ↓ 21–36% ApoB ↓ 19–28%
Stein et al. [40]	Placebo controlled RCT	10, 20 and 40 mg	132	10–17 Y (boys only)	HeFH	1 year	TC ↓ 13, 19 and 21% LDL ↓ 17%, 24 and 27% TG ↓ 4, 8 and 6% ApoB ↓ 23% (in 40 mg/d)
Claus et al. [41]	Placebo controlled RCT	20 mg for 4 weeks, then 40 mg	54	10–17 Y (girls only)	HeFH	24 weeks	TC ↓ 17–22% LDL ↓ 23–27% ApoB ↓ 20–23%

Group	Study design	Test group	N	Age	Condition	Duration	Outcomes
Pravastatin							
Knipscheer et al. [42]	Placebo controlled RCT	5, 10 and 20 mg	72	8–16 Y	FH	12 weeks	TC ↓ 24.6% LDL ↓ 32.9% ApoB ↓ 26.8% HDL ↑ 10.8%
Rosuvastatin							
Avis et al. [43]	Placebo controlled RCT	5, 10 and 20 mg	177	10–17 Y	FH	52 weeks	TC ↓ 27.1% LDL ↓ 33.9% TG ↓ 5.3% ApoB ↓ 24.2%
Braamskamp et al. [44]	Open label multicenter intention to treat analysis	5–20 mg	197	6–17 Y	HeFH	24 months	TC ↓ 32% LDL ↓ 43% TG ↓ 5% ApoB ↓ 36% Most adverse events mild
Stein et al. [45]	Placebo controlled cross over RCT	20 mg	13	7–15 Y	HoFH	24 weeks	Reduction of 22.3% LDL on rosuvastatin versus placebo with apheresis or ezetimibe
Simvastatin							
de Jongh et al. [46]	Placebo controlled RCT	10–40 mg	50	9–18 Y	FH	28 weeks	TC ↓ 30% LDL ↓ 39.8% TG ↓ 16.7% FMD improved in simvastatin group
García-de-la-Puente [47]	Placebo controlled cross over RCT	5–10 mg	25	4–17 Y	Hyperlipidemia secondary to renal disease	6 months	TC ↓ 23.3.4% LDL ↓ 33.1% TG ↓ 21%

Abbreviations: TC, total cholesterol; LDL, low-density lipoprotein cholesterol; HDL, high-density lipoprotein cholesterol; TG, triglyceride; apoB, apolipoprotein B; N, number of participants; Y, years; HoFH, familial homozygous hypercholesterolemia; HeFH, familial heterozygous hypercholesterolemia; FH, familial hypercholesterolemia; RCT, randomized control trial; TS, tanner stage; mg, milligram; T1D, Type 1 diabetes mellitus.

Table 5.
Prominent pediatric clinical trials with lipid lowering effects of statins.

1.11 Considerations for statin bioavailability

1.11.1 Factors affecting absorption

Recently, ontogenic and genetic factors have been described as potential variables influencing systemic availability of statins [49]. As statins are orally delivered, the gastric milieu and intestinal transport can have effects on the efficacy, and may have population and individual level variability in efficacy. Influx transport proteins such as OATP1A2 and OATP2B1, which are pH dependent, are shown to have an effect at the level of the enterocyte for absorption of statins [50]. Variations in MRP2 (*ABCC2* c.1446C>G), an efflux transporter has been shown to decrease the bioavailability of pravastatin [51]. Co-ingesting statins with food has also shown to have some variability in bioavailability that affects some statins more than others. For instance, absorption of fluvastatin, pravastatin and rosuvastatin is delayed when taken with food [52–55]. In contrast, package inserts of lovastatin state that levels are lower when administered under fasting conditions. Timing of food intake appears to have no effect on simvastatin.

Timing of administration has also shown to have some effect on bioavailability. This is due to multiple factors including diurnal cholesterol biosynthesis peak at nighttime and early morning and possibly the difference in gastric emptying, absorption and distribution. Reduction in both peak concentration as well as overall area under the curve (AUC) distribution have been described with evening administration of pravastatin and atorvastatin [56, 57]. Fluvastatin concentrations have been reportedly higher when dosed in the evening [58] while rosuvastatin remained unaffected [59]. Although statins are best given in the evening to coincide with the peak cholesterol biosynthesis at night, and the long-acting statins, atorvastatin and rosuvastatin, may be given any time, in clinical practice, the difference in efficacy in relation to the timing is negligible.

As with most oral medications, first pass metabolism is another factor with the potential to influence bioavailability and toxicity. Depending upon the statin, when the enterocyte is the level at which first-pass occurs, the bioavailability may be reduced, reducing toxicity but overall efficacy as well. If the first pass occurs at the level of the liver, since the hepatocytes are the primary target for the statins, a more favorable risk profile is potentially created. If the hepatocytes have more primary exposure, reduction in systemic availability and increased hepatic exposure should lead to lesser adverse effects while enhancing action at the target organ level, creating a more favorable safety profile [60].

1.11.2 Factors affecting metabolism

Of the multiple cytochromes that have been shown to have *in-vitro* capacity of metabolizing statins, CYP3A4 has been the most important, especially for simvastatin, lovastatin, and atorvastatin [61, 62]. Rosuvastatin is able to strongly inhibit CYP2C9 activity [63]. Clinically, the co-administration of CYP3A4 inhibitors like clarithromycin, erythromycin, diltiazem, itraconazole, ketoconazole, ritonavir, verapamil, goldenseal, grapefruit, etc. can lead to significant elevations in statin levels, and have the risk of higher toxicity. Inducers of CYP3A4 including phenobarbital, phenytoin, rifampicin, St. John's Wort and glucocorticoids can reduce the bioavailability of statins [64].

While considering drug interactions, concomitant administration of other lipid lowering therapy has to be kept in mind, especially for treatment of conditions such as FCH. For instance, gemfibrozil, which is used to lower TG levels, can engage with the OATP1B1-mediated transport of the statin into the hepatocyte and gut cells. It can also catalyze glucuronidation. The net effect is these interactions are a higher concentration of systemic statin level and a greater risk of adverse effects [62, 65].

1.11.3 Factors affecting elimination

Elimination can be significantly impacted by half-lives as mentioned in **Table 4**. Some statins including atorvastatin and simvastatin undergo conjugation while pravastatin, rosuvastatin, and pitavastatin do not undergo extensive conjugation. Biliary excretion of the UGT-conjugated statins occurs through—multidrug resistance 1 (MDR1; *ABCB1*), multidrug resistance-associated protein 2 (MRP2; *ABCC2*), breast cancer resistance protein (BCRP; *ABCG2*), bile salt exporting pump (BSEP; *ABCB11*) [60]. Although these efflux transporters have had *in vitro* effects, the *in vivo* effects of variants of these transporters are not well studied. Renal clearance is less significant than the biliary elimination of statins [55, 66, 67]. Of the statins, pravastatin is the most renally cleared at around 20% [68].

1.12 Adverse effects of statin therapy

Of all the classes of lipid lowering medications, statins are best tolerated with least reported adverse events [69]. The safety profile of statins has been well studied in adults. Most studies studying the safety and efficacy of statins are in children with FH. The most commonly reported side effects including muscle related adverse events and hepatic transaminase occur relatively infrequently. When statin treatment was starting to be recommended as young as 8 years of age, there were fair concerns about the effects on cognition, growth and development, metabolic rate with potential for decades of exposure to this medication.

Multiple studies have shown no adverse effects of statins on growth and sexual maturation [70]. In addressing the overall safety profile of statins, a recent meta-analysis showed that statin treatment was effective for treating FH, with a good short-term safety profile [69]. The 10- and 20-year follow-up studies on the use of statins in pediatric dyslipidemias did not report significant serious adverse events [20, 71]. There is a dearth of large long-term randomized controlled trials to establish the long-term safety issues of statins.

1.12.1 Rhabdomyolysis/myopathy

Lipophilic statins are more prone to causing myopathy as they attain greater intramuscular concentrations compared to hydrophilic statins. Pravastatin and rosuvastatin are hydrophilic, others are lipophilic. However, fluvastatin, a lipophilic statin has reportedly lower side muscle-related side effects. Non-specific muscle aches and weakness has been described with all the statins. An extensive systematic review on statin safety in adults determined rhabdomyolysis to be rare at 3 per 100,000 person-years for atorvastatin, simvastatin, lovastatin, pravastatin, and fluvastatin [72]. In children, three large systematic reviews did not find any difference between the statin group and control group for rhabdomyolysis (CK levels increased 10 fold from upper limit of normal) [69, 73, 74]. *Clinically important rhabdomyolysis* is evidence of muscle cell destruction or enzyme leakage, regardless of the CK level, considered to be causally related to a change in renal function. In practice, when CK levels are up trending and elevated to >10 upper limit of normal, with or without co-existent myoglobinuria and/or renal injury, it is recommended to stop the statin [75]. Given that this is a rare side effect, common causes including exercise, cold exposure, trauma, seizures, hypothyroidism, recent infections/myositis, autoimmune etiologies etc. need to be considered. Therapy can be commenced, preferably with a different statin when the CK levels normalize.

Statin induced myopathy is exceedingly rare in children with FH. In adults, myopathy, which includes myalgia and an increase in serum CK levels, occurs in approximately 0.1–1% of patients using statins. The risk factors associated with this are concomitant renal insufficiency, hepatic dysfunction, hypothyroidism, polypharmacy and intake of CYP3A4 inhibitors [76]. Of the reported cases, a co-existent polymorphism in SLCO1B1 resulting in decreased transport of statins into the hepatocytes, thereby increasing systemic toxicity was discovered, especially with lipophilic statins like simvastatin. Statin induced myopathy was 4.5 and 16.9 times more likely in heterozygote and homozygote carriers with this polymorphism [77].

1.12.2 Hepatic dysfunction

This is a rare side effect in statins, and in adult studies, the overall incidence of persistent transaminase elevation is considered to be about 0.5–3%. The Scandinavian Simvastatin Survival Study as well as the Heart Protection Study Collaboration group, as well as the Air Force/Texas Coronary Atherosclerosis Prevention Study, which were large randomized trials that studied simvastatin and lovastatin in large populations did not find significant differences in persistent hepatic transaminases between statin and placebo therapy in adults [78–80]. In children, three large systematic reviews did not find any difference between the statin group and control group for incidence of transaminitis (over 3-fold increase in alanine transferase or aspartate aminotransferase) [69, 73, 74].

Previously, patients receiving statins routinely measured liver function studies for monitoring transaminase elevation. In 2012, the FDA withdrew this requirement, and in practice, liver enzymes are measured as clinically needed. The examiner should inform the patient/parent to report symptoms of jaundice, malaise and fatigue as a sign of potential hepatotoxicity. In practice, if transaminase levels are found to be greater than 3 times the baseline either in symptomatic patients or during routine evaluation, the test should be repeated and other etiologies ruled out as well, given the rare incidence. During the work up process, one should consider discontinuation or dose reduction based on the presentation. Currently, the benefit of statin therapy far outweighs the risk of liver- and muscle-related adverse events.

1.12.3 Teratogenicity/need for contraception

Traditionally, animal studies have shown the potential of teratogenicity with statins due to disruption of cholesterol synthesis [81, 82]. Human studies in this regard are lacking, and the data we have so far is derived mostly from small cohort studies and case reports [83]. Contrastingly, some cohort studies did not find a significant teratogenic effect from maternal use of statins in the first trimester [84]. A meta-analysis of 6 controlled studies including a total of 618 women failed to find an increase in the risk of birth defects [85]. Many of these studies, however, were small, short term and insufficiently powered, making it difficult to generalize the results. At this time, women of childbearing age, as well as pubertal girls should be advised about concerns of teratogenicity with statin use in pregnancy, and counseled on the importance of concomitant contraceptive use.

1.12.4 Risk of type 2 diabetes mellitus (T2DM)

One of the concerning long-term side effects of statin treatment in children has been the higher risk of developing T2DM. A meta-analysis of RCTs in ~91,000 adult patients showed that statin therapy was associated with a 9% increase in the incidence of T2DM. Although there was a slightly increased risk of development of diabetes, the absolute risk as well as the comparative risk when measured against risk of coronary risk reduction was low [86]. In contrast, other studies in patients with FH treated with statins did not show a higher risk [87]. In pediatrics, the available data have been mostly reassuring, with two large 10- and 20-year follow-up studies not showing a significant increase in the incidence of T2DM when compared to the general population incidence [20, 71].

1.12.5 Concerns for non-specific effects on reduced cholesterol synthesis

Cholesterol is utilized by ubiquitously, and has a number of biological functions in other cells in the body; therefore, many non-hepatic cells also are capable of synthesizing LDL-R for uptake of cholesterol. Cholesterol is a precursor for both steroid and sex hormones. However, the use of statins has not been associated with adverse effects on the production of hormones that depend on normal sterol level availability, for instance, the adrenal hormones [74]. Fetal and neonatal cholesterol levels are lower, suggesting that an optimal homeostatic mechanism exists in which even during periods of high metabolic demand, lower levels of cholesterol are sufficient to support normal biological function [88]. Although some variations in dehydroepiandrosterone sulfate (DHEAS) and luteinizing hormone (LH) levels are reported in the literature, these differences were too small to have clinical relevance, given that the studied children did not have any growth or pubertal abnormalities [74].

2. Conclusions

Pediatric dyslipidemia could be due to monogenic, secondary or polygenic causes. Fatty plaques, the precursors of atherosclerosis and exposure to cardiovascular risk factors begin in childhood and progress into adulthood. All children with dyslipidemia benefit from diet and lifestyle modifications but the effect is limited in children with markedly elevated LDL levels. Statins are first line pharmacotherapeutic agents for elevated LDL concentrations with a favorable safety profile and robust short-term data with benefits outweighing the risks. Long-term data are needed in children to better understand the safety and efficacy of these medications.

Conflict of interest

The authors declare no conflict of interest.

Appendices and nomenclature

BP	blood pressure
BMI	body mass index
TC	total cholesterol
LDL	low density lipoprotein cholesterol
HDL	high density lipoprotein cholesterol
TG	triglyceride
AD	autosomal dominant

AR	autosomal recessive
LDL-R	LDL receptor
NHLBI	National Heart Lung and Blood Institute
NCEP	National Cholesterol Education program
USPSTF	United States Preventive Services Task Force
HoFH	familial homozygous hypercholesterolemia
HeFH	familial heterozygous hypercholesterolemia
FCH	familial combined hyperlipidemia
HMG-CoA reductase	3-hydroxy-3-methylglutaryl-coenzyme A reductase
PCSK9	proprotein convertase subtilisin/kexin type 9
apoB	apolipoprotein
ABCG	ATP-binding cassette sub-family G member
LIPA	lysosomal acid lipase type A
LPL	lipoprotein lipase
GPIHBP1	glycosylphosphatidylinositol anchored high density lipoprotein binding protein 1
LCAT	lecithin cholesterol acyl transferase
CVD	cardiovascular disease
CK	creatinine kinase

Author details

Bhuvana Sunil and Ambika Pallikunnath Ashraf*
Department of Pediatrics, Division of Endocrinology, University of Alabama, Birmingham, USA

*Address all correspondence to: aashraf@peds.uab.edu

References

[1] Benjamin EJ, Muntner P, Bittencourt MS. Heart disease and stroke statistics-2019 update: A report from the American Heart Association. Circulation. 2019;**139**(10):e56-e528

[2] Freedman DS, Khan LK, Dietz WH, Srinivasan SR, Berenson GS. Relationship of childhood obesity to coronary heart disease risk factors in adulthood: The Bogalusa Heart Study. Pediatrics. 2001;**108**(3):712-718

[3] McGill HC Jr, McMahan CA, Gidding SS. Preventing heart disease in the 21st century: Implications of the Pathobiological Determinants of Atherosclerosis in Youth (PDAY) study. Circulation. 2008;**117**(9):1216-1227

[4] Webber LS, Srinivasan SR, Wattigney WA, Berenson GS. Tracking of serum lipids and lipoproteins from childhood to adulthood. The Bogalusa Heart Study. American Journal of Epidemiology. 1991;**133**(9):884-899

[5] FOR EPOIG, CHILDREN RRI. Expert panel on integrated guidelines for cardiovascular health and risk reduction in children and adolescents: Summary report. Pediatrics. 2011;**128**(Suppl 5):S213

[6] Brown M, Goldstein J. A receptor-mediated pathway for cholesterol homeostasis. Science. 1986;**232**(4746): 34-47

[7] Ness GC, Chambers CM, Lopez D. Atorvastatin action involves diminished recovery of hepatic HMG-CoA reductase activity. Journal of Lipid Research. 1998;**39**(1):75-84

[8] Schaefer J, Schweer H, Ikewaki K, Stracke H, Seyberth H, Kaffarnik H, et al. Metabolic basis of high density lipoproteins and apolipoprotein AI increase by HMG-CoA reductase inhibition in healthy subjects and a patient with coronary artery disease. Atherosclerosis. 1999;**144**(1):177-184

[9] Martin G, Duez H, Blanquart C, Berezowski V, Poulain P, Fruchart J-C, et al. Statin-induced inhibition of the rho-signaling pathway activates PPARα and induces HDL apoA-I. The Journal of Clinical Investigation. 2001;**107**(11): 1423-1432

[10] Goldstein JL, Brown MS. Regulation of the mevalonate pathway. Nature. 1990;**343**(6257):425

[11] Cho K-J, Hill MM, Chigurupati S, Du G, Parton RG, Hancock JF. Therapeutic levels of the hydroxmethylglutaryl-coenzyme A reductase inhibitor lovastatin activate ras signaling via phospholipase D2. Molecular and Cellular Biology. 2011; **31**(6):1110-1120

[12] Labos C, Brophy JM, Smith GD, Sniderman AD, Thanassoulis G. Evaluation of the pleiotropic effects of statins. Arteriosclerosis, Thrombosis, and Vascular Biology. 2018;**38**(1):262-265

[13] Kwak B, Mulhaupt F, Myit S, Mach F. Statins as a newly recognized type of immunomodulator. Nature Medicine. 2000;**6**(12):1399

[14] Ritchie SK, Murphy EC, Ice C, Cottrell LA, Minor V, Elliott E, et al. Universal versus targeted blood cholesterol screening among youth: The CARDIAC project. Pediatrics. 2010; **126**(2):260-265

[15] Versmissen J, Oosterveer DM, Yazdanpanah M, Defesche JC, Basart DC, Liem AH, et al. Efficacy of statins in familial hypercholesterolaemia: A long term cohort study. BMJ. 2008;**337**:a2423

[16] American Academy of Pediatrics endorsement: Screen all children ages 9–11 for cholesterol. AAP News. 2011: E111111-1

[17] Grundy SM, Stone NJ, Bailey AL, Beam C, Birtcher KK, Blumenthal RS, et al. 2018 AHA/ACC/AACVPR/AAPA/ABC/ACPM/ADA/AGS/APhA/ASPC/NLA/PCNA Guideline on the Management of Blood Cholesterol: A report of the American College of Cardiology/American Heart Association Task Force on Clinical Practice Guidelines. Circulation. 2019;**139**(25): e1082-ee143

[18] Mach F, Baigent C, Catapano AL, Koskinas KC, Casula M, Badimon L, et al. 2019 ESC/EAS Guidelines for the management of dyslipidaemias: Lipid modification to reduce cardiovascular risk: The Task Force for the management of dyslipidaemias of the European Society of Cardiology (ESC) and European Atherosclerosis Society (EAS). European Heart Journal. 2020; **41**(1):111-188

[19] Bibbins-Domingo K, Grossman DC, Curry SJ, Davidson KW, Epling JW, García FA, et al. Screening for lipid disorders in children and adolescents: US Preventive Services Task Force recommendation statement. Journal of the American Medical Association. 2016;**316**(6):625-633

[20] Luirink IK, Wiegman A, Kusters DM, Hof MH, Groothoff JW, de Groot E, et al. 20-year follow-up of statins in children with familial hypercholesterolemia. New England Journal of Medicine. 2019;**381**(16): 1547-1556

[21] Nordestgaard BG, Langsted A, Mora S, Kolovou G, Baum H, Bruckert E, et al. Fasting is not routinely required for determination of a lipid profile: Clinical and laboratory implications including flagging at desirable concentration cut-points—A joint consensus statement from the European Atherosclerosis Society and European Federation of Clinical Chemistry and Laboratory Medicine. European Heart Journal. 2016;**37**(25): 1944-1958

[22] Doran B, Guo Y, Xu J, Weintraub H, Mora S, Maron DJ, et al. Prognostic value of fasting versus nonfasting low-density lipoprotein cholesterol levels on long-term mortality: Insight from the National Health and Nutrition Examination Survey III (NHANES-III). Circulation. 2014;**130**(7):546-553

[23] Eissa MA, Mihalopoulos NL, Holubkov R, Dai S, Labarthe DR. Changes in fasting lipids during puberty. The Journal of Pediatrics. 2016; **170**:199-205

[24] National Cholesterol Education Program (NCEP): Highlights of the report of the expert panel on blood cholesterol levels in children and adolescents. Pediatrics. 1992;**89**(3): 495-501

[25] Cook S, Kavey REW. Dyslipidemia and pediatric obesity. Pediatric Clinics. 2011;**58**(6):1363-1373

[26] Saland JM, Ginsberg H, Fisher EA. Dyslipidemia in pediatric renal disease: Epidemiology, pathophysiology, and management. Current Opinion in Pediatrics. 2002;**14**(2):197-204

[27] Gabriela Brenta M, Fretes O. Dyslipidemias and hypothyroidism. Pediatric Endocrinology Reviews (PER). 2014;**11**(4):390-399. PMID: 24988692

[28] Arnaldi G, Scandali VM, Trementino L, Cardinaletti M, Appolloni G, Boscaro M. Pathophysiology of dyslipidemia in Cushing's syndrome. Neuroendocrinology. 2010;**92**(Suppl 1):86-90

[29] Lanes R, Soros A, Gunczler P, Paoli M, Carrillo E, Villaroel O, et al. Growth hormone deficiency, low levels of adiponectin, and unfavorable plasma lipid and lipoproteins. The Journal of Pediatrics. 2006;**149**(3):324-329

[30] Wild R, Weedin EA, Wilson D. Dyslipidemia in pregnancy. Cardiology Clinics. 2015;**33**(2):209-215

[31] Henkin Y, Como JA, Oberman A. Secondary dyslipidemia: Inadvertent effects of drugs in clinical practice. Journal of the American Medical Association. 1992;**267**(7):961-968

[32] Yu-Poth S, Zhao G, Etherton T, Naglak M, Jonnalagadda S, Kris-Etherton PM. Effects of the National Cholesterol Education Program's Step I and Step II dietary intervention programs on cardiovascular disease risk factors: A meta-analysis. The American Journal of Clinical Nutrition. 1999;**69**(4):632-646

[33] Jones PH, Davidson MH, Stein EA, Bays HE, McKenney JM, Miller E, et al. Comparison of the efficacy and safety of rosuvastatin versus atorvastatin, simvastatin, and pravastatin across doses (STELLAR* Trial). American Journal of Cardiology. 2003;**92**(2):152-160

[34] McCrindle BW, Ose L, Marais AD. Efficacy and safety of atorvastatin in children and adolescents with familial hypercholesterolemia or severe hyperlipidemia: A multicenter, randomized, placebo-controlled trial. The Journal of Pediatrics. 2003;**143**(1):74-80

[35] Gandelman K, Glue P, Laskey R, Jones J, LaBadie R, Ose L. An eight-week trial investigating the efficacy and tolerability of atorvastatin for children and adolescents with heterozygous familial hypercholesterolemia. Pediatric Cardiology. 2011;**32**(4):433-441

[36] Canas JA, Ross JL, Taboada MV, Sikes KM, Damaso LC, Hossain J, et al. A randomized, double blind, placebo-controlled pilot trial of the safety and efficacy of atorvastatin in children with elevated low-density lipoprotein cholesterol (LDL-C) and type 1 diabetes. Pediatric Diabetes. 2015;**16**(2):79-89

[37] Langslet G, Breazna A, Drogari E. A 3-year study of atorvastatin in children and adolescents with heterozygous familial hypercholesterolemia. Journal of Clinical Lipidology. 2016;**10**(5):1153-62.e3

[38] Van Der Graaf A, Nierman MC, Firth JC, Wolmarans KH, Marais AD, De Groot E. Efficacy and safety of fluvastatin in children and adolescents with heterozygous familial hypercholesterolaemia. Acta Paediatrica. 2006;**95**(11):1461-1466

[39] Lambert M, Lupien P-J, Gagné C, Lévy E, Blaichman S, Langlois S, et al. Treatment of familial hypercholesterolemia in children and adolescents: Effect of lovastatin. Pediatrics. 1996;**97**(5):619-628

[40] Stein EA, Illingworth DR, Kwiterovich J, Peter O, Liacouras CA, Siimes MA, et al. Efficacy and safety of lovastatin in adolescent males with heterozygous familial hypercholesterolemia A randomized controlled trial. Journal of the American Medical Association. 1999;**281**(2):137-144

[41] Clauss SB, Holmes KW, Hopkins P, Stein E, Cho M, Tate A, et al. Efficacy and safety of lovastatin therapy in adolescent girls with heterozygous familial hypercholesterolemia. Pediatrics. 2005;**116**(3):682-688

[42] Knipscheer H, Boelen C, Kastelein J, Van Diermen D, Groenemeijer B, Van Den Ende A, et al. Short-term efficacy and safety of pravastatin in 72 children with familial hypercholesterolemia. Pediatric Research. 1996;**39**(5):867

[43] Avis HJ, Hutten BA, Gagné C, Langslet G, McCrindle BW, Wiegman A, et al. Efficacy and safety of rosuvastatin therapy for children with familial hypercholesterolemia. Journal

of the American College of Cardiology. 2010;**55**(11):1121-1126

[44] Braamskamp MJ, Langslet G, McCrindle BW, Cassiman D, Francis GA, Gagné C, et al. Efficacy and safety of rosuvastatin therapy in children and adolescents with familial hypercholesterolemia: Results from the CHARON study. Journal of Clinical Lipidology. 2015; **9**(6):741-750

[45] Stein EA, Dann EJ, Wiegman A, Skovby F, Gaudet D, Sokal E, et al. Efficacy of rosuvastatin in children with homozygous familial hypercholesterolemia and association with underlying genetic mutations. Journal of the American College of Cardiology. 2017; **70**(9):1162-1170

[46] de Jongh S, Lilien MR, Jos op't Roodt J, Stroes ES, Bakker HD, Kastelein JJ. Early statin therapy restores endothelial function in children with familial hypercholesterolemia. Journal of the American College of Cardiology. 2002;**40**(12):2117-2121

[47] García-de-la-Puente S, Arredondo-García JL, Gutiérrez-Castrellón P, Bojorquez-Ochoa A, Maya ER, Pérez-Martínez MDP. Efficacy of simvastatin in children with hyperlipidemia secondary to kidney disorders. Pediatric Nephrology. 2009;**24**(6):1205-1210

[48] Association AD. 12. Children and adolescents: Standards of medical care in diabetes—2018. Diabetes Care. 2018; **41**(Supplement 1):S126-S136

[49] Wagner J, Leeder JS. Pediatric pharmacogenomics: A systematic assessment of ontogeny and genetic variation to guide the design of statin studies in children. Pediatric Clinics. 2012;**59**(5):1017-1037

[50] Nozawa T, Imai K, Nezu J, Tsuji A, Tamai I. Functional characterization of pH-sensitive organic anion transporting polypeptide OATP-B in human. The Journal of Pharmacology and Experimental Therapeutics. 2004; **308**(2):438-445

[51] Shirasaka Y, Suzuki K, Nakanishi T, Tamai I. Intestinal absorption of HMG-CoA reductase inhibitor pravastatin mediated by organic anion transporting polypeptide. Pharmaceutical Research. 2010;**27**(10):2141-2149

[52] Pan HY, DeVault AR, Brescia D, Willard DA, McGovern ME, Whigan DB, et al. Effect of food on pravastatin pharmacokinetics and pharmacodynamics. International Journal of Clinical Pharmacology, Therapy, and Toxicology. 1993;**31**(6): 291-294

[53] Radulovic LL, Cilla DD, Posvar EL, Sedman AJ, Whitfield LR. Effect of food on the bioavailability of atorvastatin, an HMG-CoA reductase inhibitor. Journal of Clinical Pharmacology. 1995;**35**(10): 990-994

[54] Shang D, Deng S, Yao Z, Wang Z, Ni X, Zhang M, et al. The effect of food on the pharmacokinetic properties and bioequivalence of two formulations of pitavastatin calcium in healthy Chinese male subjects. Xenobiotica. 2016;**46**(1): 34-39

[55] Smith HT, Jokubaitis LA, Troendle AJ, Hwang DS, Robinson WT. Pharmacokinetics of fluvastatin and specific drug interactions. American Journal of Hypertension. 1993;**6**(11 Pt 2):375s-382s

[56] Triscari J, Rossi L, Pan HY. Chronokinetics of pravastatin administered in the PM compared with AM dosing. American Journal of Therapeutics. 1995;**2**(4): 265-268

[57] Cilla DD Jr, Gibson DM, Whitfield LR, Sedman AJ. Pharmacodynamic effects and

pharmacokinetics of atorvastatin after administration to normocholesterolemic subjects in the morning and evening. Journal of Clinical Pharmacology. 1996; **36**(7):604-609

[58] Fauler G, Abletshauser C, Erwa W, Loser R, Witschital K, Marz W. Time-of-intake (morning versus evening) of extended-release fluvastatin in hyperlipemic patients is without influence on the pharmacodynamics (mevalonic acid excretion) and pharmacokinetics. International Journal of Clinical Pharmacology and Therapeutics. 2007;**45**(6): 328-334

[59] Martin PD, Mitchell PD, Schneck DW. Pharmacodynamic effects and pharmacokinetics of a new HMG-CoA reductase inhibitor, rosuvastatin, after morning or evening administration in healthy volunteers. British Journal of Clinical Pharmacology. 2002;**54**(5): 472-477

[60] Wagner J, Abdel-Rahman SM. Pediatric statin administration: Navigating a frontier with limited data. Journal of Pediatric Pharmacology and Therapeutics. 2016;**21**(5):380-403

[61] Prueksaritanont T, Ma B, Yu N. The human hepatic metabolism of simvastatin hydroxy acid is mediated primarily by CYP3A, and not CYP2D6. British Journal of Clinical Pharmacology. 2003;**56**(1):120-124

[62] Prueksaritanont T, Gorham LM, Ma B, Liu L, Yu X, Zhao JJ, et al. In vitro metabolism of simvastatin in humans [SBT]identification of metabolizing enzymes and effect of the drug on hepatic P450s. Drug Metabolism and Disposition. 1997;**25**(10):1191-1199

[63] Sakaeda T, Fujino H, Komoto C, Kakumoto M, Jin JS, Iwaki K, et al. Effects of acid and lactone forms of eight HMG-CoA reductase inhibitors on CYP-mediated metabolism and MDR1-mediated transport. Pharmaceutical Research. 2006;**23**(3):506-512

[64] Neuvonen PJ, Niemi M, Backman JT. Drug interactions with lipid-lowering drugs: Mechanisms and clinical relevance. Clinical Pharmacology and Therapeutics. 2006; **80**(6):565-581

[65] Shitara Y, Hirano M, Sato H, Sugiyama Y. Gemfibrozil and its glucuronide inhibit the organic anion transporting polypeptide 2 (OATP2/ OATP1B1: SLC21A6)-mediated hepatic uptake and CYP2C8-mediated metabolism of cerivastatin: Analysis of the mechanism of the clinically relevant drug-drug interaction between cerivastatin and gemfibrozil. Journal of Pharmacology and Experimental Therapeutics. 2004;**311**(1):228-236

[66] Stern RH, Yang BB, Horton M, Moore S, Abel RB, Olson SC. Renal dysfunction does not alter the pharmacokinetics or LDLholesterol reduction of atorvastatin. Journal of Clinical Pharmacology. 1997;**37**(9): 816-819

[67] Martin PD, Warwick MJ, Dane AL, Hill SJ, Giles PB, Phillips PJ, et al. Metabolism, excretion, and pharmacokinetics of rosuvastatin in healthy adult male volunteers. Clinical Therapeutics. 2003;**25**(11):2822-2835

[68] Everett DW, Chando TJ, Didonato GC, Singhvi SM, Pan HY, Weinstein SH. Biotransformation of pravastatin sodium in humans. Drug Metabolism and Disposition. 1991; **19**(4):740-748

[69] Vuorio A, Kuoppala J, Kovanen PT, Humphries SE, Tonstad S, Wiegman A, et al. Statins for children with familial hypercholesterolemia. Cochrane Database of Systematic Reviews. 2017;**7**

[70] Humphries SE, Cooper J, Dale P, Ramaswami U. The UK paediatric

familial hypercholesterolaemia register: Statin-related safety and 1-year growth data. Journal of Clinical Lipidology. 2018;**12**(1):25-32

[71] Kusters DM, Avis HJ, de Groot E, Wijburg FA, Kastelein JJ, Wiegman A, et al. Ten-year follow-up after initiation of statin therapy in children with familial hypercholesterolemia. Journal of the American Medical Association. 2014;**312**(10):1055-1057

[72] Law M, Rudnicka AR. Statin safety: A systematic review. The American Journal of Cardiology. 2006;**97**(8):S52-S60

[73] Arambepola C, Farmer AJ, Perera R, Neil HA. Statin treatment for children and adolescents with heterozygous familial hypercholesterolaemia: A systematic review and meta-analysis. Atherosclerosis. 2007;**195**(2):339-347

[74] Avis HJ, Vissers MN, Stein EA, Wijburg FA, Trip MD, Kastelein JJ, et al. A systematic review and meta-analysis of statin therapy in children with familial hypercholesterolemia. Arteriosclerosis, Thrombosis, and Vascular Biology. 2007;**27**(8):1803-1810

[75] Thompson PD, Clarkson PM, Rosenson RS. An assessment of statin safety by muscle experts. American Journal of Cardiology. 2006;**97**(8a): 69c-76c

[76] Rosenson RS. Current overview of statin-induced myopathy. The American Journal of Medicine. 2004; **116**(6):408-416

[77] Link E, Parish S, Armitage J, Bowman L, Heath S, Matsuda F, et al. SLCO1B1 variants and statin-induced myopathy—A genomewide study. The New England Journal of Medicine. 2008;**359**(8):789-799

[78] Downs JR, Clearfield M, Weis S, Whitney E, Shapiro DR, Beere PA, et al. Primary prevention of acute coronary events with lovastatin in men and women with average cholesterol levels: Results of AFCAPS/TexCAPS. Air Force/Texas Coronary Atherosclerosis Prevention Study. Journal of the American Medical Association. 1998; **279**(20):1615-1622

[79] Randomised trial of cholesterol lowering in 4444 patients with coronary heart disease: The Scandinavian Simvastatin Survival Study (4S). Lancet. 1994;**344**(8934):1383-1389

[80] MRC/BHF Heart Protection Study of cholesterol lowering with simvastatin in 20,536 high-risk individuals: A randomised placebo-controlled trial. Lancet. 2002;**360**(9326):7-22

[81] Edison RJ, Muenke M. Mechanistic and epidemiologic considerations in the evaluation of adverse birth outcomes following gestational exposure to statins. American Journal of Medical Genetics Part A. 2004;**131**(3):287-298

[82] Godfrey LM, Erramouspe J, Cleveland KW. Teratogenic risk of statins in pregnancy. Annals of Pharmacotherapy. 2012;**46**(10): 1419-1424

[83] Edison RJ, Muenke M. Central nervous system and limb anomalies in case reports of first-trimester statin exposure. The New England Journal of Medicine. 2004;**350**(15):1579-1582

[84] Bateman BT, Hernandez-Diaz S, Fischer MA, Seely EW, Ecker JL, Franklin JM, et al. Statins and congenital malformations: Cohort study. BMJ: British Medical Journal. 2015;**350**:h1035

[85] Zarek J, Koren G. The fetal safety of statins: A systematic review and meta-analysis. Journal of Obstetrics and Gynaecology Canada. 2014;**36**(6): 506-509

[86] Sattar N, Preiss D, Murray HM, Welsh P, Buckley BM, de Craen AJ,

et al. Statins and risk of incident diabetes: A collaborative meta-analysis of randomised statin trials. The Lancet. 2010;**375**(9716):735-742

[87] Besseling J, Kastelein JJ, Defesche JC, Hutten BA, Hovingh GK. Association between familial hypercholesterolemia and prevalence of type 2 diabetes mellitus. Journal of the American Medical Association. 2015; **313**(10):1029-1036

[88] Woollett L, Heubi JE. Fetal and neonatal cholesterol metabolism. In: Feingold KR, Anawalt B, Boyce A, Chrousos G, Dungan K, Grossman A, et al., editors. Endotext. South Dartmouth (MA): MDText.com, Inc.; 2000

Chapter 6

Pharmacokinetic Aspects of Statins

Lucía Cid-Conde and José López-Castro

Abstract

Statins are the most used therapeutic group in the treatment of hypercholesterolemia and reduce the risk of cardiovascular events and mortality. Long prescription periods and their pharmacokinetic characteristics increase the possibility of interactions, especially at the metabolism level. Simvastatin, lovastatin, and atorvastatin are metabolized by CYP3A4 isoenzymes, so they will have more significant interactions than fluvastatin, pitavastatin, and rosuvastatin that require CYP2C9. The main interactions are with macrolides, azole antifungals, antiretrovirals, platelet antiaggregants, anticoagulants, oral antidiabetics, calcium channel blockers, immunosuppressants, and other hypolipidemic agents, among others. A review of all medications that are taken by patients treated with statins should be performed at each medical consultation and during all healthcare transitions.

Keywords: drug interactions, metabolism, isoenzymes CYP3A4, rhabdomyolysis, hypolipidemic drugs

1. Introduction

As a consequence of the variability in their origin, statins have notable differences; however, their pharmacodynamic similarities allow them to be grouped together for study. As for the mechanism of action, its effects and the clinical consequences of its use, there is an important group congruence already well known.

Nowadays, seven statins are commonly used: lovastatin (first licensed in 1987), simvastatin (1988), pravastatin (1991), fluvastatin (1994), atorvastatin (1997), rosuvastatin, and pitavastatin (2003). Cerivastatin, approved in 1998, was subsequently withdrawn from the world market due to a high risk of rhabdomyolysis.

They are the most therapeutic group used in the treatment of hypercholesterolemia and most have been shown to reduce the risk of events and cardiovascular mortality; however, the long prescription periods of these drugs and their pharmacokinetic characteristics increase the possibility of drug interactions [1].

2. Statins pharmacokinetics

2.1 Absorption

The interaction of statins at the level of absorption can translate into a decrease in the absorption of the drug by a change in pH, a variation in the speed of intestinal motility or the formation of complexes and/or chelates.

All currently marketed statins are absorbed orally in a variable range (between 30% for lovastatin and 35% for pravastatin), so the influence of intake at the time of administration is very important to achieve an effect adequate therapeutic [2].

The absorption of a drug can be reduced, delayed, or increased by food consumption, as they share many physiological mechanisms and coincide with numerous organs. This is why the medication schedule is so important in these drugs. In general, all statins reduce their absorption in the presence of food so that their administration is usually at night, before bedtime, and without food, although there are some exceptions. When pravastatin is administered with food, its bioavailability is reduced by approximately 35% compared to that obtained in its administration before meals. This bioavailability reduction is also observed for fluvastatin, both water soluble, so it is recommended to space its administration with respect to meals at least 4 hours. As for atorvastatin, it seems that a meal with a medium fat content may slightly reduce its absorption, while with simvastatin, it does not seem that this fact is relevant. Unlike the previous ones, the administration of lovastatin after a meal increases its plasma concentration by 50% compared to the fasting state. Therefore, it is recommended that lovastatin be taken with food. As for the most recent statins, rosuvastatin and pitavastatin, rosuvastatin has an absorption in which plasma concentrations are reached at approximately 5 hours after oral administration. The total bioavailability is approximately 20%. Rosuvastatin, unlike its group mates, can be taken at any time of the day, its absorption being the same with both food and without food.

Likewise, pitavastatin is widely absorbed by 80%, without interacting with food. There is no accumulation due to repeat multiple doses; therefore, the single dose is accepted.

2.2 Distribution

Plasma protein binding is variable, but in general, it is very high. Except for 50% of pravastatin, all are above 95%. The tissue distribution is wide, crossing the blood-brain and placental barriers, even passing into breast milk. No clinically important interactions have been described by displacement of statins from their binding to plasma proteins. However, the fact that statins could be displaced by another drug is a fact that must always be taken into consideration and studied to discover a possible case.

The hepatic specificity of these drugs is determined by their degree of lipophilicity and by the presence of organic anion transport proteins (OATPs) that allow more hydrophilic statins such as pitavastatin, pravastatin, and rosuvastatin to enter the hepatocyte. The lipophilic statins (atorvastatin, fluvastatin, lovastatin, and simvastatin) can enter directly in cells. On the other hand, some statins can inhibit P-glycoprotein (multidrug resistance protein), a drug-carrying protein in the cell, so they could lead to drug interactions. Lovastatin and simvastatin are ingested as lipophilic lactone prodrugs, whereas other statins are administered as active acid forms.

2.3 Metabolism

Statins are metabolized by CYP450 isoenzymes, with the exception of pravastatin, which is metabolized in the cellular cytosol by sulfation. In addition, they present gastrointestinal and hepatic first-pass metabolism. There are differences in metabolism with respect to gender and age, but not enough to modify the doses in the absence of other pathologies (**Table 1**).

Enzyme	Statin Substrates	Inhibitors	Inducers
CYP2C9	Fluvastin, rosuvastatin (also CYP2C19)	Amiodarone, capecitabine, etravirine, fluconazole, fluvoxamine, fluvastatin, ketoconazole, metronidazole, miconazole, oxandrolone, sulfamethoxazole/ trimethoprim, voriconazole, zafirlukast	Carbamazepine, phenobarbital, phenytoin rifampin
CYP3A4	Atorvastatin, lovastatin, simvastatin	Amiodarone,amlodipine, aprepitant, atorvastatin, bicalutamide, cilostazol, cimetidine, ciprofloxacin, clarithromycin, conivaptan, cyclosporine, diltiazem, erythromycin, fluconazole, fluoxetine, fluvoxamine, grapefruit juice, imatinib, isoniazid, itraconazole, ketoconazole, mibefradil, midazolam, nefazodone, nilotinib, posaconazole, protease inhibitors, ranolazine, sertraline, tacrolimus, telithromycin, ticagrelor, tricyclic antidepressants, verapamil, voriconazole	Aprepitant, bosentan, carbamazepine, cyclophosphamide, corticosteroids, efavirenz, modafnil, nafcillin, nevirapine, phenytoin, pioglitazone, phenobarbital, rifampin, St. John's wort
P-gp	Atorvastatin, lovastatin, pitavastatin, simvastatin	Amiodarone, atorvastatin, azithromycin, captopril, carvedilol, cimetidine, clarithromycin, colchicine, conivaptan, cyclosporine, diltiazem, dipyridamole, dronedarone, erythromycin, felodipine, grapefruit juice, itraconazole, ketoconazole, lovastatin, mefloquine, nicardipine, omeprazole, protease inhibitors, quinidine, ranolazine, reserpine, sertraline, simvastatin, tacrolimus, verapamil	Carbamazepine, phenytoin rifampin, St. John's wort
OATP1B1	Atorvastatin, pitavastatin, pravastatin, rosuvastatin, simvastatin	Carbamazepine, clarithromycin, cyclosporine, erythromycin, gemfibrozil, protease inhibitors, roxithromycin, rifampin, sildenafil, sacubitril, telithromycin	Unknown
OATP1B3	Fluvastatin, pravastatin, rosuvastatin	Clarithromycin, cyclosporine, erythromycin, rifampin, roxithromycin, rifampin, sacubitril, telithromycin	Unknown

CYP: cytochrome P; OATP: Organic Anion-Transporting Polypeptide; P-gp: permeability glycoprotein

Table 1.
Common P-gp substrates, inhibitors, and inducers associated with the CYP450 enzymes affecting statin metabolism [42].

CYP450 metabolizes a high percentage of drugs, especially the CYP3A4 isoenzyme (about 36%). The main factors that affect the metabolism by this route are enzyme induction, enzyme inhibition, and genetic polymorphisms.

Enzymatic inducer is that medication that stimulates the synthesis and/or activity of a CYP450 isoenzyme, usually CYP3A4. This produces a stimulation of the metabolism of both the inducing drug itself (self-induction) and the drug administered concomitantly, in this case the statin, so it would reduce more rapidly its plasma concentrations. A reduction in plasma concentrations results in a lower effect of the hypolipemiant drug. In the case of having to administer the two medications, it would be necessary to perform blood concentration tests and, if necessary, increase the dose of statin. The most frequent enzyme inducers are rifampicin, rifabutin, phenobarbital, carbamazepine, phenytoin, nevirapine, efavirenz, troglitiazone, polyglitazone, or St. John's wort (Hipérico).

Enzymatic inhibitor is that medication that, administered together with the statin, inhibits a CYP450 isoenzyme. This produces a decrease in statin metabolism, increasing its plasma concentrations, and can cause adverse effects. The most potent and frequent enzyme inhibitors are protease inhibitors such as ritonavir (potent antiretroviral used precisely because of its inhibitory role in potentiation pharmacokinetics) and some macrolides such as erythromycin, proton pump inhibitors such as omeprazole, azole antifungals such as ketoconazole or itraconazole, or the juice of Grapefruit, among many others.

The metabolites can be hydroxylated, omega or beta-oxidized, methylated, or glucuronized derivatives, whose pharmacological activity is highly variable.

Therefore, the spectrum of clinical effectiveness is wide, from lovastatin or simvastatin, which are really pharmacologically inactive lactones and that carry out their pharmacological activity through their metabolites, to fluvastatin, which has practically inactive metabolites.

Simvastatin and lovastatin undergo significant CYP3A4 metabolism and atorvastatin undergoes a lesser amount as one of its minor metabolic pathways.

This is in contrast to fluvastatin, pitavastatin, and rosuvastatin, which require CYP2C9. Because CYP3A4 is the most common enzyme involved in drug metabolism, simvastatin and lovastatin will have more interactions that will likely require intervention [2].

Thus, state-of-the-art statins, rosuvastatin and pitavastatin, are minimally metabolized by CYP450 isoenzymes and by P-glycoprotein. This causes them to have a lower probability of interactions. Pitavastatin, on the other hand, has minimal hepatic metabolism due to the first step (enterohepatic circulation). It is practically not metabolized; it is mainly eliminated by bile route; and its renal excretion as an active drug is minimal (less than 2%). The main metabolic pathway of pitavastatin is lactonization/glucuronidation. Rosuvastatin is also not metabolized by cytochrome CYP3A4; it uses CYP2C9 and CYP2C19 but it does so in a very low percentage [3].

P-glycoprotein (P-gp) is responsible for the intestinal and biliary elimination of some of the statins such as pravastatin or atorvastatin.

2.4 Excretion

The amount of statin that is excreted in its unchanged form through renal elimination is small. The overall dependence of statin metabolites on renal elimination is modest, with pravastatin being the highest at 20% and atorvastatin being the lowest at <2%.

Fluvastatin, lovastatin, pravastatin, and simvastatin have a relatively short half-life (less than 5 hours). These medications are optimally dosed at night or given as an extended-release formulation to maximize the effect (fluvastatin or lovastatin). By contrast, pitavastatin (12 hours), atorvastatin (14 hours), and rosuvastatin (between 15 and 30 hours) have longer half-lives and can be dosed at any time of the day.

Statins are also excreted into bile and feces as a means of drug elimination. This excretion is facilitated by OATPs. Similar to CYP450, there are several subtypes of OATP that can affect the elimination of rosuvastatin and pitavastatin [2].

The drug interactions with statins may sometimes be attributable to decreased drug excretion, especially in patients with impaired glomerular filtration rate, and are related to the extent the statin is renally excreted. This potential issue is limited with atorvastatin, which has the least amount of renal excretion (<2%), but may be a consideration for other statins that have a higher degree of renal excretion (pitavastatin, pravastatin, rosuvastatin, simvastatin) (**Table 2**).

	Absorption		Distribution		Metabolism			Excretion	
	Bioavailability %	T_{max} h	Protein binding %	Lipophilicity	Major P450 Hepatic Enzyme	Prodrug	Active metabolites	Excretion Biliary Renal %	$T_{1/2}$ h
Atorvastatin	12	1-2	>98	Yes	CYP3A4	No	Yes	<1% <2%	14
Fluvastatin	24	<1	>98	Yes	CYP2C9	No	No	>90% 6%	3
Lovastatin	<5	2-4	>95	Yes	CYP3A4	Yes	Yes	83% 10%	2-3
Pitavastatin	>60	1	>99	Yes	CYP2C9	No	No	79% 15%	12
Pravastatin	18	1-1,5	50	No	Non-CYP	No	No	71% 20%	1-3
Rosuvastatin	20	3-5	90	No	CYP2C9	No	Minimal	90% 10%	19
Simvastatin	<	4	>95	Yes	CYP3A4	Yes	Yes	58% 13%	2

CYP: cytochrome P; t1/2: drug half-life; Tmax: time that a drug is present at the maximum concentration in serum.

Table 2.
Pharmacokinetic properties of statins [2].

3. Interactions

The long prescription periods of these drugs and their pharmacokinetic characteristics already exposed, increase the possibility of drug interactions. The most frequent adverse effects are headache, gastrointestinal discomfort, cramps, and asymptomatic elevation of transaminases, among others. The most important safety problem is myopathy, which can progress to rhabdomyolysis and death of the patient (**Table 3**).

3.1 Drug-drug interactions

HMG-CoA reductase inhibitors have different pharmacokinetic profiles, which may affect potential drug interactions.

3.1.1 Antiplatelet agents

There is controversy between the interaction of clopidogrel with statins motivated mainly by differences in the design and method of the studies.

So, no effect of atorvastatin or any statin on antiplatelet activity of single dose of clopidogrel found in prospective study of 25 patients taking atorvastatin, 25 patients taking other statin, and 25 patients taking no statin [4].

This administration of CYP3A4-metabolized statins in clopidogrel treated patients does not induce any changes in the conversion of clopidogrel into its active thiol form and therefore neither has a quantitatively nor clinically relevant influence on clopidogrel efficacy [5].

Several randomized clinical trials (RCTs) compare the results of patients in whom clopidogrel was associated and a statin metabolized by CYP3A4 (atorvastatin, lovastatin, simvastatin); with those treated with statins not metabolized by CYP3A4 (fluvastatin and pravastatin). Patients treated with atorvastatin had similar rates of bleeding and complications, without any interaction being checked [6]. In other trials, the inhibition of platelet aggregation was similar when fluvastatin, pravastatin, or atorvastatin was associated with clopidogrel [7].

In a cohort study conducted in 10,491 patients who were prescribed clopidogrel, when comparing 43.5% of the patients who were associated with atorvastatin, with whom a non-CYP3A4 statin was associated, or with the group that did not receive statin, there was no increase in possible side effects [8].

A clinical trial of 50 patients comparing the association of clopidogrel-acetylsalicylic acid with that of atorvastatin-clopidogrel, after a “bypass” of the coronary artery, shows that the combination with atorvastatin further increased platelet inhibition and, consequently, the antiaggregant effect would be greater than the association with acetylsalicylic acid [9].

Clinical trials have evaluated pharmacokinetic interactions of ticagrelor coadministered with atorvastatin, simvastatin, or lovastatin. They have shown an increase in Cmax (maximum concentration) and AUC (area under the curve) of atorvastatin, simvastatin, or lovastatin as a result of CYP3A4 inhibition by ticagrelor. However, these changes were not statistically significant [10]. The dose of simvastatin and lovastatin should not exceed 40 mg daily when prescribed with ticagrelor. There were no clinically significant interactions when ticagrelor is used in combination with pravastatin, fluvastatin, pitavastatin, or rosuvastatin, and no dosing restrictions were needed. No clinically significant drug interactions have been reported with prasugrel in combination with statins.

Interacting Agent		Statin	Effect	Magnitude	Recommendation
Antiarrhythmic agent	Amiodarone	Simvastatin Lovastatin	Increased statin exposure/increased risk for muscle-related toxicity	Minor	Combination therapy may be considered
	Dronedarone	Lovastatin Simvastatin	Decreased metabolis of statin leading to increased concentrations increased statin exposure/increased risk for muscle-related toxicity	Moderate	Combination may be considered
	Digoxin	Atorvastatin	Increased levels of digoxin	Minor	Combination is reasonable
Azole antifungals (fluconazole, itraconazole)		Simvastatin Lovastatin Atorvastatin Fluvastatin	Increased statin exposure/increased risk for muscle-related toxicity	Severe	Combination is potentially harmful
Anticoagulants (warfarin)		Simvastatin Lovastatin Fluvastatin Rosuvastatin	Increase INR/ potential for increased bleeding	Variable	Combination therapy is useful
Antiretroviral	All protease inhibitors	Simvastatin Lovastatin	Increased statin exposure/increased risk for muscle-related toxicity	Severe	Combination is potentially harmfull
	Saquinavir/ritonavir Nelfinavir	Atorvastatin	Increased statin exposure/increased risk for muscle-related toxicity	Moderate	Administer lower dose of atorvastatin
	Nelfinavir	Pravastatin	Decreased metabolism of statin	Moderate	Combination is reasonable, adjust dose pravastatin
	Lopinavir/ritonavir Atazanavir/ritonavir	Rosuvastatin	Increased statin exposure	Moderate	Combination is reasonable, adjust dose rosuvastatin
	Efavirenz	Simvastatin Lovastatin Atorvastatin Pravastatin	Decreased metabolis of statin	Moderate	Combination is reasonable, adjust dose statin
Calcium channel blockers	Dihydropyridine calcium antagonist (amlodipine)	Lovastatin Simvastatin	Increased statin exposure/increased risk for muscle-related toxicity	Minor	Combination therapy may be considered
	Non-dihydropyridine calcium antagonists (verapamil)	Lovastatin Simvastatin Atorvastatin	Decreased metabolis of statin leading to increased concentrations increased risk of muscle-related toxicity	Moderate	Combination may be considered
Colchicine		Atorvastatin Fluvastatin Lovastatin Pitavastatin Pravastatin Rosuvastatin Simvastatin	Increased statin or colchicine exposure/increased risk for muscle-related toxicity	Variable	Combination may be considered
Fibrates (fenofibrate)		Atorvastatin Fluvastatin Lovastatin Pitavastatin Rosuvastatin Simvastatin	Potential increase in muscle-related toxicity	Insignificant	Combination is reasonable
Gemfibrozil		Atorvastatin Pitavastatin Rosuvastatin	Decreased metabolis of statin leading to increased concentrations /increased risk for muscle-related toxicity	Minor/ moderate	Combination may be considered
		Lovastatin Pravastatin			Combination should be avoided
		Simvastatin			Avoid combination
Inmunosuppressants (cyclosporine/tacrolimus/ everolimus/sirolimus)		Atorvastatin Fluvastatin Pravastatin Rosuvastatin	Increased statin exposure through multiple mechanisms Increased risk for	Severe	Combination therapy may be considered
		Simvastatin Lovastatin Pitavastatin	muscle-related toxicity		Combination is potentially harmfull
Macrolides (clarithromycin, erythromycin, telithromycin)		Simvastatin Lovastatin Atorvastatin	Increased statin exposure/increased risk for muscle-related toxicity	Severe	Combination is potentially harmful
Ranolazine		Lovastatin Simvastatin	Increased statin exposure/increased risk for muscle-related toxicity	Minor	Combination therapy may be considered
Ticagrelor		Atorvastatin	Increased statin exposure/increased risk for muscle-related toxicity	Minor	Combination is reasonable
		Lovastatin Simvastatin	Decreased metabolis of statin leading to increased concentrations /increased risk for muscle-related toxicity	Moderate	Combination may be considered

Table 3.
Statin interactions [7, 8, 13, 23, 25, 37, 39].

3.1.2 Anticoagulants

The warfarin and statin interaction information is limited; however, the case reports show a possible effect on coagulation, especially with fluvastatin or rosuvastatin [11] (for its potent inhibitory effect on CYP2C9) and lovastatin (possibly due to the displacement of protein binding). Other statins, except pravastatin, could have interactions, by inhibition of warfarin or acenocoumarol metabolism, or by displacement of protein binding.

Several studies neither have demonstrated significant interaction between warfarin-pitavastatin [12] and warfarin-atorvastatin [13], nor have shown clinically significant drug interactions with statins and new anticoagulants such as dabigatran, apixaban, rivaroxaban, and edoxaban.

The use of statins with warfarin as combination therapy is useful when clinically indicated. It is advisable to monitor the international normalized ratio (INR) more closely when a statin is started or changed in dose. The impact on the INR appears lowest for pitavastatin and atorvastatin [14].

3.1.3 Oral antidiabetics

It has been shown that statins and metformin reduce inflammation and oxidative stress. These results show an additional cardioprotective effect, as a direct action mechanism or through its pleiotropic effects. That is why patients with type II diabetes mellitus often take metformin and statins together to control the risk of cardiovascular disease and glucose metabolism. Metformin shows beneficial effects on both dyslipidemia and glycemic control and it has been shown to reduce the risk of cardiovascular disease. While statins can have an additional beneficial effect on the risk of cardiovascular disease, the combined treatment with both medications seems be a good therapeutic option [15].

The prescription of statins and dipeptidyl peptidase 4 (DPP-4) inhibitors is becoming common in patients with type 2 diabetes mellitus and hyperlipidemia. Several mechanisms have been proposed to describe the interaction between the two, ranging from the effects of sitagliptin on renal excretion of statins to interaction at the level of liver metabolism [16]. A case report of simvastatin-induced rhabdomyolysis in the presence of sitagliptin proposed that the nephrotoxicity of sitagliptin led to reduced renal excretion of simvastatin [17].

However, a clinical trial that studied the effects of sitagliptin on the pharmacokinetics of simvastatin in 12 healthy human subjects aged 18–45 years, both male and female, showed no effect on simvastatin metabolism [18]. The authors did not recommend dose adjustment, when simvastatin was coadministered with sitagliptin. Similarly, another study in 10 patients found no effects of the use of simvastatin on the pharmacokinetics of sitagliptin, and no dose adjustment was recommended for any of the drugs [19].

In a case report of rhabdomyolysis induced by lovastatin and sitagliptin, the authors suggested an interaction between statin and sitagliptin at the CYP3A4 level as the cause. They claimed that because both are metabolized by CYP3A4, when coadministered, they can compete for the same enzyme, resulting in a higher serum statin concentration, which leads to statin-induced rhabdomyolysis [20]. Two other case reports of rhabdomyolysis with atorvastatin and sitagliptin had similar suggestions, indicating that sitagliptin leads to an increase in serum concentration of atorvastatin through its effects on liver metabolism by CYP3A4 rather than on renal excretion. A thorough review of the literature suggests that atorvastatin and sitagliptin are not prone to drug pharmacokinetic interactions, either separately or in a fixed combination of drugs.

Statins that can cause rhabdomyolysis by interaction with sitagliptin are lovastatin, atorvastatin, and simvastatin as they are all metabolized by CYP3A4. This interaction is not described with statins that are not metabolized by CYP3A4 such as pravastatin, rosuvastatin, pitavastatin, and fluvastatin.

When exenatide (10 mcg twice daily) was administered concomitantly with a single dose of lovastatin (40 mg), the values of AUC and Cmax of lovastatin decreased approximately 40 and 28%, respectively, and the Tmax (maximum concentration time required) was delayed about 4 hours. In the 30-week placebo-controlled clinical trials, the concomitant use of exenatide and hydroxymethylglutaryl coenzyme A (HMG CoA) inhibitors was not associated with consistent changes in lipid profiles. Although no dose adjustment is required, possible changes in LDL-C or total cholesterol should be taken into account. The lipid profile should be evaluated regularly. Liraglutide did not modify the general exposure of atorvastatin to a clinically significant degree following the administration of a single dose of 40 mg of atorvastatin; therefore, no dose adjustment of atorvastatin is necessary when administered with liraglutide. There was a 38% decrease in atorvastatin Cmax, and the average Tmax was delayed 1–3 hours with liraglutide [3].

3.1.4 Azole antifungals

Azole antifungals are inhibitors of the CYP3A4 isoenzyme although itraconazole is more potent than fluconazole. When administered concomitantly with statins, a metabolic block can occur with an increase in plasma concentrations of the latter and the possibility of unwanted effects [21].

There are case reports of myopathy and rhabdomyolysis due to the simultaneous use of simvastatin or atorvastatin with itraconazole and fluconazole. A study that evaluated the effect of itraconazole on the pharmacokinetics of lovastatin in 12 healthy volunteers showed an increase in Cmax of 13 times (range 10–23 times) and 20 times in the AUC of the active metabolite of lovastatin [22].

On the other hand, two randomized double-blind, two-phase, cross-sectional studies conducted to evaluate the effect of fluconazole on plasma concentrations of fluvastatin and pravastatin showed an increase in the AUC and Cmax of fluvastatin by 84 and 44%, respectively; while no significant changes in pravastatin levels were documented.

Itraconazole increased by 15 times the AUC and the Cmax of lovastatin; likewise, simvastatin showed a significant increase in the Cmax and AUC of the acid form (β-hydroxy acid) by 17 and 19 times, respectively. Therefore, the concomitant use of lovastatin and simvastatin with itraconazole should be avoided by the potential increase in toxicity on skeletal muscle. On the other hand, the use of itraconazole with fluvastatin or pravastatin did not generate significant changes in the levels of these statins. Similarly, the combination of fluconazole with rosuvastatin generated an increase in the AUC and Cmax of rosuvastatin without clinical relevance [23].

3.1.5 Antiretroviral agents (ARV)

The use of lipid-lowering drugs in patients with HIV/AIDS is increasingly frequent, due to the increase in life expectancy of this group of patients, a situation that is associated with the presentation of other health problems, such as increased cardiovascular risk, accelerated biological aging, chronic inflammatory process, and prolonged exposure to medications ARV [24].

Metabolism of protease inhibitors (PI) and non-nucleoside reverse transcriptase inhibitors (NNRTIs) is mainly due to CYP3A4 inhibition. Pravastatin, due to its metabolic mechanism of sulfation, is of choice in patients treated with PI (except darunavir), although in some cases, it may be necessary to increase the dose of pravastatin, for example, with nelfinavir or ritonavir. The use of simvastatin, lovastatin, and atorvastatin (except pravastatin, fluvastatin, and rosuvastatin) should be avoided in patients with PI treatment, especially with ritonavir, atazanavir, saquinavir, or nelfinavir [25]. However, it is necessary to keep in mind that the combination of rosuvastatin with lopinavir/ritonavir caused an increase in the AUC and Cmax of rosuvastatin of 2.1 and 4.7 times, respectively. AUC and Cmax of rosuvastatin were increased by 213 and 600% when atazanavir/ritonavir was administered.

Efavirenz decreased the AUC of atorvastatin, simvastatin, and pravastatin by 43, 58, and 40%, respectively. It is recommended to carry out a closer follow-up and if necessary, adjust the dose of statins [26].

3.1.6 Calcium channel blockers

Non-dihydropyridine calcium antagonists (verapamil and diltiazem) have a significant increase in AUC and Cmax when coadministered with simvastatin, lovastatin, and atorvastatin, due to inhibition of P-gp activity (decreased efflux) or enzymatic inhibition of CYP3A4. Lovastatin increased the AUC and Cmax of verapamil by 62.8 and 32.1%; while verapamil AUC was increased by 42.8% in the presence of atorvastatin. On the other hand, simvastatin increased its AUC and Cmax 2.6 and 4.6 times, respectively, due to the use of verapamil. Additionally, there are reports of cases of rhabdomyolysis due to the combination verapamil, cyclosporine, and simvastatin. Diltiazem can cause an increase in Cmax by 3.6 times and the AUC by 5 times of simvastatin and 3.5 times of lovastatin; effect that is not evident in the case of pravastatin [27]. It should be noted that although the inhibitory effect of diltiazem on simvastatin increases the pharmacological effect of statins, an increased risk of myopathy is also observed. According to the above, there is a report of cases of myopathy and/or rhabdomyolysis with doses equal to and greater than 20 mg of simvastatin or atorvastatin. A dose adjustment is recommended in patients treated with verapamil and simvastatin (maximum 20 mg) or lovastatin (maximum 40 mg). Pravastatin, for which no relevant interactions have been described at the CYP450 level, could be an alternative for patients who need treatment with calcium channel blockers that interfere with CYP3A4.

Dihydropyridine calcium antagonist (amlodipine) produces an increase in the Cmax and AUC of simvastatin and atorvastatin, without significant effects on lipid or blood pressure and combination therapy may be considered [28]. The separate administration of at least 4 hours of simvastatin and amlodipine minimizes the occurrence of this interaction [29, 30].

3.1.7 Antiarrhythmic agents

Amiodarone is an inhibitor of CYP3A4 (irreversibly) and P-gp (reversible), causing interactions when used concomitantly with statins metabolized by CYP450 or substrates of the P-gp. There have been reports of toxicity between amiodarone and statins that are CYP3A4 substrates, particularly simvastatin. Thus, a 75% increase in AUC and Cmax of simvastatin has been demonstrated when co-administered with amiodarone. However, there are no significant pharmacokinetic interactions between amiodarone and pravastatin [31].

Muscle-related toxicity was the most commonly reported adverse event with combination therapy (77%). The percentages of simvastatin and atorvastatin adverse events reported in which amiodarone was concomitantly used were 1.0 and 0.7%, respectively. By contrast, the percentage of pravastatin adverse events in which amiodarone was used was only 0.4%. Patients on simvastatin-amiodarone combination therapy were more likely to be hospitalized and were on a higher statin dose compared with atorvastatin-amiodarone-treated patients. No dose adjustment for rosuvastatin, pravastatin, fluvastatin, and pitavastatin is necessary when coadministered concomitantly with amiodarone.

Additionally, no dose adjustments are recommended for atorvastatin because data suggest that severe interactions with amiodarone are less likely to occur than with other statins metabolized via CYP3A4 (simvastatin and lovastatin). Lovastatin should not exceed 40 mg daily when prescribed in combination with amiodarone and simvastatin, and should be limited to no more than 20 mg daily. On the basis of pharmacokinetic and observational data and adverse events reported in randomized, controlled trials, combination therapy with amiodarone and rosuvastatin, atorvastatin, pitavastatin, fluvastatin, or pravastatin is reasonable.

Coadministration of amiodarone and dronedarone with either lovastatin or simvastatin may be considered. When used in combination with amiodarone, the dose of lovastatin should not exceed 40 mg daily and the dose of simvastatin should not exceed 20 mg daily. There are no known clinically significant interactions between dronedarone and other statins.

Digoxin is not dependent on the CYP450 system because it is not known to induce or inhibit any of these enzymes. Metabolism of digoxin is primary by gut bacteria. In a study that included 24 healthy volunteers, the addition of atorvastatin 80 mg to digoxin resulted in an average increase of 20% in the Cmax of digoxin and an average 15% increase in the AUC of digoxin [32]. However, lower doses of atorvastatin (10 mg) combined with digoxin did not alter the pharmacokinetics of digoxin. Atorvastatin appears to be the only statin that is reported to have this interaction. The mechanism is not fully understood but may be mediated by an impact of atorvastatin on the intestinal secretion of digoxin medicated by the P-gp efflux transporter, resulting in an increased digoxin absorption. The existence of alternatives to atorvastatin, such as fluvastatin, pravastatin, and rosuvastatin, which do not affect P-gp, may be of choice in patients treated with digoxin.

3.1.8 Immunosuppressants

The combination of statins with calcineurin inhibitors (cyclosporine and tacrolimus), due to its inhibitory effect of CYP3A4, inhibitor of OATPB1 and be substrates of P-gp, could cause an increase in serum statin levels and the risk of myopathy and rhabdomyolysis, especially at high doses of statins.

There are reports of cases of rhabdomyolysis with different statins, except fluvastatin and, to a lesser extent, pravastatin. In the case of simvastatin, AUC increases up to 20 times and the effect is enhanced by the use of other CYP3A4 enzymatic inhibitors. On the other hand, in the case of atorvastatin, cases of rhabdomyolysis present without alterations the pharmacokinetics of cyclosporine. Cyclosporine is associated with an increase in AUC and Cmax of rosuvastatin by 7.1 and 10.6 times, respectively.

There is evidence of the safety and effectiveness of fluvastatin in transplant patients treated with cyclosporine. This effect could be due to the fact that fluvastatin, compared to other statins, has a shorter elimination half-life, a greater capacity for protein binding and less circulating active metabolites. In the case of pravastatin, this drug does not accumulate significantly in plasma in patients receiving immunosuppression with cyclosporine, and with rosuvastatin, cyclosporine increased the AUC of this statin by 7.1 times.

Limited data exist on tacrolimus and statin interactions. One open-label evaluation of 13 healthy volunteers suggested that after 4 days of therapy with atorvastatin 40 mg daily, 2 doses of tacrolimus had no impact on the atorvastatin pharmacokinetics [33].

In case reports, the use of sirolimus in combination with statins has been associated with muscle-related toxicity, including rhabdomyolysis. Only one randomized, open-label, three-way crossover, single-dose study in 24 healthy volunteers has suggested that everolimus had no effect on the AUC of atorvastatin 20 mg or pravastatin 20 mg [34].

The combination therapy of cyclosporine, tacrolimus, everolimus or sirolimus with lovastatin, simvastatin, and pitavastatin is potentially harmful and should be avoided. The combination of cyclosporine, tacrolimus, everolimus, or sirolimus with daily dose of fluvastatin, pravastatin and rosuvastatin may be considered and should be limited to 40, 20, and 5 mg daily, respectively. The dose of atorvastatin >10 mg daily when coadministered with cyclosporine, tacrolimus, everolimus, or sirolimus is not recommended without close monitoring of creatinine kinase and signs or symptoms of muscle-related toxicity. The combination of fluvastatin-rapamycin has been linked to the appearance of rhabdomyolysis.

3.1.9 Macrolides

Macrolides, especially clarithromycin, erythromycin, and telithromycin, are the most potent inhibitors of the CYP3A4 isoenzyme, followed by the weak inhibitor, roxithromycin, and finally, azithromycin. CYP3A4 is an isoenzyme that metabolizes simvastatin, lovastatin, and atorvastatin, which increases their plasma concentrations and the risk of myotoxicity. Rosuvastatin, fluvastatin, and pravastatin are not significantly affected by this interaction. Of all macrolides, azithromycin can be used with statins. Erythromycin increased the Cmax of simvastatin (in its lactone form) by 3.4 times, the AUC by 6.2 times and its acid-hydroxy acid form by 3.9 times. Erythromycin increased Cmax and AUC of atorvastatin by 37.7 and 32.5%, respectively. The effect is attributed to decreased metabolism of statins, inhibition of intestinal P-gp, and decreased bile secretion.

In general, case reports of rhabdomyolysis are available due to the interaction between simvastatin and clarithromycin, between lovastatin and erythromycin, and between clarithromycin and azithromycin [35]. A study that evaluated the effect of azithromycin and clarithromycin on the pharmacokinetics of atorvastatin showed that clarithromycin increases AUC and Cmax by 82 and 56%, respectively; meanwhile, there were no significant changes with azithromycin.

3.1.10 Interactions between lipid lowering agents

Some patients may require the combination of several lipid lowering agents, the statin-fibrate association being the most common. However, the greater hypolipidemic effect is accompanied by an increased risk of myopathy, especially with gemfibrozil, due to its inhibitory effect on glucuronidation of statins, increasing the concentrations of the latter.

Gemfibrozil increases the AUC of simvastatin by 35% and the AUC of simvastatin in its acid form by 135% and of lovastatin acid by 280%. Therefore, there is a report of cases of rhabdomyolysis and kidney disease, due to the combination of gemfibrozil with simvastatin, atorvastatin, and lovastatin.

In addition, gemfibrozil increases the AUC of rosuvastatin by 1.88 times and its Cmax by 2.21 times [36]. Gemfibrozil had only a modest effect when administered with pitavastatin in 24 subjects with an increase of 45% in the AUC [37]. Metabolism is only a minor pathway for pitavastatin via CYP2C9, which is unaffected by gemfibrozil. Fluvastatin transport in hepatocytes via the OATP transporters is potently inhibited by gemfibrozil [38]. However, in at least 1 study of 17 subjects, no significant difference was observed in the AUC and Cmax in a comparison of the gemfibrozil-fluvastatin combination and gemfibrozil alone.

Related to this interaction, it is important to note that fenofibrate is considered more suitable than gemfibrozil, which is supported in studies showing the absence of interaction of fenofibrate with pravastatin, simvastatin, and atorvastatin.

However, fenofibrate may increase rosuvastatin plasma levels and there is a case report of renal failure in a patient taking this combination.

The combination of gemfibrozil with lovastatin, pravastatin, and simvastatin is potentially harmful and should be avoided. Although gemfibrozil interacts with atorvastatin, pitavastatin, and rosuvastatin, the result is only a minor increase in statin concentrations, and the combination may be considered if clinically indicated. Fluvastatin may be used in combination with gemfibrozil without any specific dose limitations, and this particular statin does not interact with gemfibrozil.

Combination therapy with fenofibrate/fenofibric acid and any statin is reasonable when clinically indicated.

Ezetimibe is well tolerated and does not interact with fluvastatin, lovastatin, rosuvastatin, or simvastatin. However, cases of myopathy have been reported in patients due to the combination ezetimibe and atorvastatin.

3.1.11 Antidepressants

Although coadministration of statins and antidepressants is likely, given the association between depression and many chronic diseases, the prevalence of clinically relevant interactions between them is not well-documented.

With the exception of atorvastatin and fluvastatin, which inhibit the activity of CYP3A4 and CYP2C9, respectively, most statins do not appear to be inhibitors or inducers of the main drug metabolizing enzymes. On the other hand, some antidepressants act as inhibitors of several CYPs and, therefore, may impair the elimination of statins metabolized through these isoforms. Based on this knowledge, it can be anticipated that concomitant use of nefazodone or fluvoxamine, potent or moderate CYP3A4 inhibitors, respectively, with atorvastatin, lovastatin, or simvastatin should increase the plasma concentrations of these statins.

Statin metabolism may be susceptible to OATP inhibition by imipramine, nortriptyline, and amitriptyline, with a possible increase in drug concentration. Atorvastatin, a CYP3A4 inhibitor, can act on the metabolism of tricyclic antidepressants (excluding nortriptyline). Also, an interaction between imipramine (a P-gp substrate) and statins (P-gp inhibitors) could be hypothesized.

Fluvoxamine is the only moderate CYP3A4 inhibitor, and may be associated with an increased risk of interactions if administered with atorvastatin, lovastatin, and simvastatin. While the potential interaction between fluoxetine and statins has not been investigated in humans, experimental evidence in animal models found that the combination of simvastatin with fluoxetine may enhance anxiolytic and antidepressant properties. Both fluvoxamine and fluoxetine act as moderate inhibitors of CYP2C9 activity and, in theory, can increase plasma concentrations of fluvastatin, which is metabolized primarily through this isoform. However, the magnitude of this interaction would probably be below the threshold of clinical importance. Due to the theoretical risk of a metabolic interaction, lower doses of atorvastatin, lovastatin, and simvastatin may be indicated in patients treated with fluvoxamine. On the other hand, it is unlikely that the pharmacokinetics of pitavastatin and rosuvastatin, minimally metabolized by CYP2C9, may be significantly affected by the coadministration of fluvoxamine and fluoxetine.

In the case of joint administration of selective inhibitors reuptake serotonins (SSRIs) with statins, escitalopram, citalopram, and sertraline appear to be safe with all statins.

Coadministration with statins metabolized through CYP3A4 (atorvastatin, simvastatin, and lovastatin) or, to a lesser extent, fluvastatin through CYP2D6, could lead to a potentially competitive inhibition. However, there are no clinical or in vitro studies available on possible interactions between serotonin and norepinephrine reuptake inhibitor (SNRI)/norepinephrine reuptake inhibitor (NRI)/vortioxetine and statins. Venlafaxine and duloxetine have two main metabolic pathways: CYP2D6 and CYP3A4 or CYP2D6 and CYP1A2, respectively.

There are no studies on the coadministration of specific noradrenergic and serotonergic antidepressants (NaSSA), mirtazapine coadministered with statins. According to in vitro studies, mirtazapine is metabolized by CYP1A2, CYP2D6 and, to a lesser extent by CYP3A4 and inhibits CYP2D6 and CYP1A2 with negligible potency. Therefore, there is a low probability of interactions.

With respect to the norepinephrine-dopamine reuptake inhibitor (NDRI), bupropion is a moderate CYP2D6 inhibitor and is metabolized by CYP2D6. Considering the lacking of in vitro and in vivo pharmacokinetics studies and the metabolic pathway of statins, with only fluvastatin metabolized to a lesser extent by CYP2D6 and the high rate of renal excretion (>85%), the intereactions pharmacokinetics are no probable [39].

3.1.12 Other drugs

The joint use of simvastatin with *erlotinib* or *imatinib* has been related to cases of rhabdomyolysis. In addition, imatinib (CYP3A4 inhibitor) increases the AUC of simvastatin 3.5 times [40].

With the concomitant use of simvastatin and *pazopanib*, an increase in the incidence of ALT elevations has been documented, so simvastatin treatment should be discontinued when these alterations are observed. In addition, it cannot be ruled out that pazopanib affects the pharmacokinetics of other statins (atorvastatin, fluvastatin, and rosuvastatin). This potential for interaction and morbidity in cancer patients can be minimized by the use of pravastatin, instead of simvastatin, since this drug is excreted by the kidneys and has no significant metabolism via CYP3A4.

The interaction of *Rifampicin* with pravastatin is contradictory, on the one hand in one study, rifampin increased the AUC of pravastatin by 2 times; while another, in healthy volunteers, showed that rifampicin decreases plasma statin levels by 40%. With atorvastatin, rifampin decreases the AUC of atorvastatin by 80%. In the case of simvastatin, the decrease reaches 87%. On the other hand, with rosuvastatin, the effect was minor and was not considered clinically relevant.

Cholestyramine: there is possible reduction of plasma levels of statins, by fixation to the resin in the intestinal lumen and lipid-lowering activity, although clinical practice seems to indicate otherwise. It is recommended to administer the statin 1 hour before or 4 hours after the resin.

Sildenafil: there is a report of myopathy with rosuvastatin and a case of rhabdomyolysis with simvastatin.

Ciprofloxacin (weak CYP3A4 inhibitor): there is a report of rhabdomyolysis with simvastatin.

Efalizumab: there is a case report of rhabdomyolysis with pravastatin.

Danazol: it is a moderate androgen receptor agonist and a partial progestogenic agonist. It is able to inhibit the metabolism of some statins by increasing their plasma concentrations. Cases of myopathy and rhabdomyolysis have been described. Likewise, a case of acute pancreatitis was published in an 80-year-old patient treated with this combination of drugs. Although documented cases affect simvastatin and lovastatin, it is advisable to exercise caution with any statin administered in conjunction with danazol and control the occurrence of muscle symptoms.

Risperidone and simvastatin: risperidone inhibits the oxidative metabolism of statin and increases its toxicity with a risk of rhabdomyolysis. Muscle pain and weakness, with increased creatin kinase, have been reported in a patient with simvastatin 30 mg/day, 12 days after taking risperidone 1 mg/24 h.

In patients taking *ranolazine,* the use of statins, whose metabolism is highly dependent on CYP3A4 as simvastatin or lovastatin, should be limited due to the risk of rhabdomyolysis [3].

3.2 Drug-food interactions

There are phytotherapeutic agents that can interact with medications. St. John's wort is a CYP3A4 enzyme inducer, while grapefruit juice is an enzyme inhibitor.

Some studies show a decrease in statin concentrations and, therefore, their effectiveness when St. John's wort is administered with rosuvastatin, atorvastatin, or simvastatin. The effect is not observed for pravastatin. It is recommended to avoid grapefruit juice with lovastatin and simvastatin; avoid large quantities of grapefruit just if taking atorvastatin (increases in area-under-the-curve to 2.5-fold have been reported with consumption of ≥750 mL to 1.2 L per day). In the case of lovastatin, grapefruit juice causes a 12-fold increase in Cmax and 15-fold increase in AUC; on the other hand, for the acid form of lovastatin, the increase in Cmax was 4 times, and in AUC, it was 5 times. In the case of orange juice, its administration has been linked to a significant increase of pravastatin AUC in healthy volunteers [2].

Red yeast rice is a popular over-the-counter treatment for hyperlipidemia. Red yeast rice has varying amounts of monacolin K (similar to lovastatin). The products are not standardized and no red yeast rice product should be administered to a patient taking a prescribed statin.

Licorice (*Glycyrrhiza glabra* L., Licorice) in vitro has shown a slight inhibition of CYP3A4 and CYP2D6. Some cases of muscular alteration with increased creatin kinase and, in some cases, rhabdomyolysis have been reported in patients taking high amounts. The risk may increase when associated with drugs that cause muscle toxicity, such as statins, so their combination should be avoided [41].

3.3 Influence of genetic variations in the pharmacokinetic profile of the statins

The activity of the CYP3A4 and CYP2C9 isoenzymes has great interindividual variability as a result of their genetic polymorphism. SLCO1B1 polymorphisms (gene encoding the organic anion transport polypeptide, OATP1B1) can cause variability in statin plasma levels. OATP1B1 affects the hepatic uptake of statins, where statins are going to be metabolized and exert their action at the intracellular level. A reduced activity of OATP1B1 may decrease their efficacy and increase their plasma concentrations, with the consequent risk of muscle toxicity.

Thus, the Genome Wide Association Study (GWAS) studied 300,000 polymorphisms in patients treated with statins and who had presented myopathies in front of a control group with statins and who had not presented myopathies. The conclusions reached were: patients who presented the C521T > C polymorphism of the SLCO1B1 gene (also encoded as SLCO1B1* 5) should not receive treatment with statins, since they have a high risk of suffering from myalgias or myopathy after a few months of treatment; patients with polymorphisms of the CYP2C9 gene that conditions a poor metabolizer (PM) phenotype of the CYP2C9 enzyme (although they do not present mutations in the SLCO1B1 gene) will eliminate fluvastatin less efficiently and may have myopathies (administration of other types of statins is recommended); simvastatin, atorvastatin, and lovastatin are eliminated by cytochrome CYP3A4 and CYP3A4 polymorphisms that induce poor metabolizers (PM) have not been found, but it must be taken into account that many drugs are potent CYP3A4 inhibitors and a comedication with these statins could induce myopathies due to drug interaction. The application of genetic information to individualize pharmacological treatments to maximize efficacy and avoid adverse events, or pharmacogenetics, is an important component of precision medicine [42].

4. Conclusions

A review of all medications that are treated by patients treated with statins should be performed at each medical consultation and during all healthcare transitions within a health system so that drug interactions can be identified early, evaluated, and properly managed, implementing adjustments of dose, changing to another safer statin or discontinuing when necessary. A thorough understanding of the pharmacokinetics of statins and other concomitantly administered medications is paramount to ensure patient safety.

Conflict of interest

The authors declare no conflict of interest.

Author details

Lucía Cid-Conde[1] and José López-Castro[2*]

1 Pharmaceutical Specialist in Hospital Pharmacy, University Hospital Complex of Ourense, Ourense, Spain

2 Internal Medicine Department Hospital Público de Monforte, Lugo, Spain

*Address all correspondence to: jose.lopez.castro@sergas.es

References

[1] Yan MM, Wu SS, Ying YQ, Lu N, Zhong MK. Safety assessment of concurrent statin treatment and evaluation of drug interactions in China. SAGE Open Medicine. 2018;**6**:1-9

[2] Wiggins BS, Saseen JJ, Page RL, Reed BN, Sneed K, Kostis JB, et al. Recommendations for management of clinically significant drug-drug interactions with statins and select agents used in patients with cardiovascular disease. Circulatión. 2016;**134**(21):e468-e495

[3] Kellick KA, Bottorff M, Toth PP. A clinician's guide to statin drug-drug interactions. Journal of Clinical Lipidology. 2014;**8**:S30-S46

[4] Serebruany VL, Midei MG, Malinin AI, Oshrine BR, Lowry DR, Sane DC, et al. Absence of interaction between atorvastatin or other statins and clopidogrel: Results from the interaction study. Archives of Internal Medicine. 2004;**164**(18):2051-2057

[5] Siepmann T, Heinke D, Kepplinger J, Barlinn K, Gehrisch S, Grählert X, et al. Interaction of clopidogrel and statins in secondary prevention after cerebral ischaemia—A randomized, double-blind, double-dummy crossover study. British Journal of Clinical Pharmacology. 2014;**78**(5):1058-1066

[6] Han YL, Zhang ZL, Li Y, Wang SL, Jing QM, Wang ZL, et al. Comparison on long-term effects of atorvastatin or pravastatin combined with clopidogrel for patients undergoing coronary stenting: A randomized controlled trial. Zhonghua Yi Xue Za Zhi. 2009A;**89**(32): 2240-2244

[7] Wenaweser P, Eshtehardi P, Abrecht L, Zwahlen M, Schmidlin K, Windecker S, et al. A randomised determination of the effect of fluvastatin and atorvastatin on top of dual antiplatelet treatment on platelet aggregation after implantation of coronary drug-eluting stents. The EFA-trial. Thrombosis and Haemostasis. 2010;**104**(3):554-562

[8] lagojevic A, Delaney JA, Lévesque LE, Dendukuri N, Boivin JF, Brophy JM. Investigation of an interaction between statins and clopidogrel after percutaneous coronary intervention: A cohort study. Pharmacoepidemiology and Drug Safety. 2009;**18**(5):362-369

[9] Tetik S, Ak K, Isbir S, Eksioglu-Demiralp E, Arsan S, Iqbal O, et al. Clopidogrel provides significantly greater inhibition of platelet activity than aspirin when combined with atorvastatin after coronary artery bypass grafting: A prospective randomized study. Clinical and Applied Thrombosis/Hemostasis. 2010;**16**(2):189-198

[10] Teng R, Mitchell PD, Butler KA. Pharmacokinetic interaction studies of co-administration of ticagrelor and atorvastatin or simvastatin in healthy volunteers. European Journal of Clinical Pharmacology. 2013;**69**:477-487

[11] Simonson SG, Martin PD, Mitchell PD, Lasseter K, Gibson G, Schneck DW. Effect of rosuvastatin on warfarin pharmacodynamics and pharmacokinetics. Journal of Clinical Pharmacology. 2005;**45**:927-934

[12] Yu CY, Campbell SE, Zhu B, Knadler MP, Small DS, Sponseller CA, et al. Effect of pitavastatin vs. rosuvastatin on international normalized ratio in healthy volunteers on steadystate warfarin. Current Medical Research and Opinion. 2012;**28**:187-194

[13] Stern R, Abel R, Gibson GL, Besserer J. Atorvastatin does not alter the anticoagulant activity of warfarin. Journal of Clinical Pharmacology. 1997;**37**:1062-1064

[14] Guidoni CM, Camargo HPM, Obreli-Neto PR, Girotto E, Pereira LRL. Study of warfarin utilization in hospitalized patients: Analysis of possible drug interactions. International Journal of Clinical Pharmacy. 2016;**38**: 1048-1051

[15] Van Stee MF, De Graaf AA, Groen AK. Actions of metformin and statins on lipid and glucose metabolism and possible benefit of combination therapy. Cardiovascular Diabetology. 2018;**17**(1):94

[16] Bhome R, Penn H. Rabdomiólisis precipitada por una interacción farmacológica sitagliptina-atorvastatina. Diabetic Medicine. 2012;**29**(5):693-694

[17] Kao DP, Kohrt HE, Kugler J. Insuficiencia renal y rabdomiólisis asociadas con el uso de sitagliptina y simvastatina. Diabetic Medicine. 2008;**25**(10):1229-1230

[18] Bergman AJ, Cote J, Maes A, et al. Efecto de sitagliptina sobre la farmacocinética de simvastatina. Journal of Clinical Pharmacology. 2009;**49**(4):483-488

[19] Cerra M, Luo WL, Li SX, et al. Los efectos de la simvastatina en la farmacocinética de sitagliptina. Journal of Population Therapeutics and Clinical Pharmacology. 2012;**19**(3):e356-e360

[20] DiGregorio RV, Pasikhova Y. Rhabdomyolysis caused by a potential sitagliptin-lovastatin interaction. Pharmacotherapy. 2009;**29**(3):352-356

[21] Eljaaly K, Alshehri S. An updated review of interactions of statins with antibacterial and antifungal agents. Journal of Translational Science. 2017;**3**(3):1-4

[22] Tiessen RG, Lagerwey HJ, Jager GJ, Sprenger HG. Drug interaction caused by communication problems. Rhabdomyolysis due to a combination of itraconazole and simvastatin. Nederlands Tijdschrift voor Geneeskunde. 2010;**154**:A762

[23] Cooper KJ, Martin PD, Dane AL, Warwick MJ, Schneck DW, Cantarini MV. The effect of fluconazole on the pharmacokinetics of rosuvastatin. European Journal of Clinical Pharmacology. 2002;**58**:527-531

[24] Robert SR, Colantonio LD, Burkholder GA, Chen L, Muntner P. Trends in utilization of statin therapy and contraindicated statin use in HIV--infected adults treated with antiretroviral therapy from 2007 through 2015. Journal of the American Heart Association. 2018;**7**(24):1-18

[25] Giraldo NA, Amariles P, Gutiérrez FJ, Monsalve M, Faus MJ. Interacciones medicamentosas en pacientes infectados con el VIH: aproximación para establecer y evaluar su relevancia clínica: actualización 2009. Farmacia Hospitalaria. 2010;**3**(4):90-93

[26] Gerber JG, Rosenkranz SL, Fichtenbaum CJ, Vega JM, Yang A, Alston BL, et al. AIDS Clinical Trials Group A5108 team. Effect of efavirenz on the pharmacokinetics of simvastatin, atorvastatin, and pravastatin: Results of AIDS Clinical Trials Group 5108 study. Journal of Acquired Immune Deficiency Syndromes. 2005;**39**:307-312

[27] Hu M, Mak VW, Tomlinson B. Simvastatin-induced myopathy, the role of interaction with diltiazem and genetic predisposition. Journal of Clinical Pharmacy and Therapeutics. 2011;**36**:419-425

[28] Nishio S, Watanabe H, Kosuge K, Uchida S, Hayashi H, Ohashi K. Interaction between amlodipine and simvastatin in patients with hypercholesterolemia and hypertension. Hypertension Research. 2005;**28**:223-227

[29] Park CG, Lee H, Choi JW, Lee SJ, Kim SH, Lim HE. Non-concurrent dosing attenuates the pharmacokinetic interaction between amlodipine and simvastatin. International Journal of Clinical Pharmacology and Therapeutics. 2010;**48**:497-503

[30] Zhou Y-T, Yu L-S, Zeng S, Huang Y-W, Xu H-M, Zhou Q. Pharmacokinetic drug-drug interactions between 1,4-dihydropyridine calcium channel blockers and statins: Factors determining interaction strength and relevant clinical risk management. Therapeutics and Clinical Risk Management. 2014;(10):17-26

[31] Becquemont L, Neuvonen M, Verstuyft C, Jaillon P, Letierce A, Neuvonen PJ, et al. Amiodarone interacts with simvastatin but not with pravastatin disposition kinetics. Clinical Pharmacology and Therapeutics. 2007;**81**(5):679-684

[32] Boyd RA, Stern RH, Stewart BH, Wu X, Reyner EL, Zegarac EA, et al. Atorvastatin coadministration may increase digoxin concentrations by inhibition of intestinal P-glycoprotein-mediated secretion. Journal of Clinical Pharmacology. 2000;**40**:91-98

[33] Lemahieu WP, Hermann M, Asberg A, Verbeke K, Holdaas H, Vanrenterghem Y, et al. Combined therapy with atorvastatin and calcineurin inhibitors: no interactions with tacrolimus. American Journal of Transplantation. 2005;**5**:2236-2243

[34] Basic-Jukic N, Kes P, Bubic-Filipi L, Vranjican Z. Rhabdomyolysis and acute kidney injury secondary to concomitant use of fluvastatin and rapamycin in a renal transplant recipient. Nephrology, Dialysis, Transplantation. 2010;**25**:2036. author reply 2036-2037

[35] Molden E, Andersson KS. Simvastatin-associated rhabdomyolysis after coadministration of macrolide antibiotics in two patients. Pharmacotherapy. 2007;**27**:603-607

[36] Bergman E, Matsson EM, Hedeland M, Bondesson U, Knutson L, Lennernäs H. Effect of a single gemfibrozil dose on the pharmacokinetics of rosuvastatin in bile and plasma in healthy volunteers. Journal of Clinical Pharmacology. 2010;**50**:1039-1049

[37] Mathew P, Cuddy T, Tracewell WG, Salazar D. An open-label study on the pharmacokinetics (PK) of pitavastatin (NK-104) when administered concomitantly with fenofibrate or gemfibrozil in healthy volunteers. Clinical Pharmacology and Therapeutics. 2004;**75**:33

[38] Noé J, Portmann R, Brun ME, Funk C. Substrate-dependent drugdrug interactions between gemfibrozil, fluvastatin and other organic anion-transporting peptide (OATP) substrates on OATP1B1, OATP2B1, and OATP1B3. Drug Metabolism and Disposition. 2007;**35**:1308-1314

[39] Palleria C, Roberti R, Iannone LF, Tallarico M, Barbieri MA, Vero A, et al. Clinically relevant drug interactions between statins and antidepressants. Journal of Clinical Pharmacy and Therapeutics. 2019. DOI: 10.1111/jcpt.13058

[40] Weeraputhiran M, Sundermeyer M. Rhabdomyolysis resulting from pharmacologic interaction between erlotinib and simvastatina. Clinical Lung Cancer. 2008;**4**(9):232-234

[41] Vaquero MP, Sánchez Muniz FJ, Jiménez Redondo S, Prats Oliván P, Higueras FJ, Bastida S. Major diet-drug interactions affecting the kinetic characteristics and hypolipidaemic properties of statins. Nutrición Hospitalaria. 2010;**25**(2):193-206

[42] Maggo SDS, Kennedy MA, Clark DWJ. Clinical implications of pharmacogenetic variation on the effects of statins. Drug Safety. 2011;**34**:1-19